Facial Nerve Palsy - A Practitioner's Guide

Edited by Pratap Sanchetee,
Kirti Sachdeva and R. Rajeshwari

Published in London, United Kingdom

Facial Nerve Palsy - A Practitioner's Guide
http://dx.doi.org/10.5772/intechopen.102253
Edited by Pratap Sanchetee, Kirti Sachdeva and R. Rajeshwari

Contributors
Leniza Mingazova, Elena Karpova, Olga Ratmirovna Orlova, Ada Artemenko, Mario Alberto Garcia-Ramirez, Wendy Liliana Martinez Angeles, Orfil González-Reynoso, Gregorio Guadalupe Carbajal Arizaga, Alaz Cirak, Serdar Nasir, Lok Yan Joanne Cheng, Tai Hong Andrew Lung, Shu Yan Ng, Pratap Sanchetee

First published in London, United Kingdom, 2022 by IntechOpen
IntechOpen is the global imprint of INTECHOPEN LIMITED, registered in England and Wales, registration number: 11086078, 5 Princes Gate Court, London, SW7 2QJ, United Kingdom

British Library Cataloguing-in-Publication Data
A catalogue record for this book is available from the British Library

Additional hard and PDF copies can be obtained from orders@intechopen.com

Facial Nerve Palsy - A Practitioner's Guide
Edited by Pratap Sanchetee, Kirti Sachdeva and R. Rajeshwari
p. cm.
Print ISBN 978-1-83969-158-4
Online ISBN 978-1-83969-159-1
eBook (PDF) ISBN 978-1-83969-196-6

Meet the editors

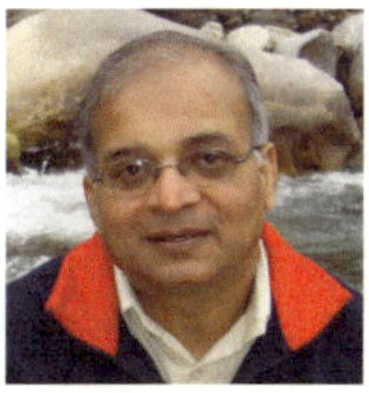

Dr. Pratap Sanchetee graduated from Dr. SN Medical College, Jodhpur in 1970, and received his MD in medicine and therapeutics from the University of Rajasthan in 1974, and DM (Neurology) from the Postgraduate Institute of Medical Education & Research (PGIMER), Chandigarh in 1985. He served in India's armed forces as a physician and neurologist for 24 years, retiring as Lt Col in 1998. From 1994 to 1998 he was also an associate professor at the Armed Forces Medical College, Pune. Since 1998, he has worked in clinical practice in neurology at various hospitals in Jodhpur and at Guwahati Assam. He has been a visiting professor, Ph.D. supervisor, and advisor at Jain Visva Bharti University (JVBI) and Bhagwan Mahaveer International Research Centre (BMIRC), Ladnun, Rajasthan, since 2009. He is the Director of Research at the Spiritual Training Research Foundation (STRF), Mumbai. His areas of active interest are the mind as an interface between soul and body; meditation and the brain; and the delivery of neurology care in society. Dr. Sanchetee has edited six books and published 120 original papers, chapters, and review articles in national and international journals. For over 10 years he was associated with the tropical neurology subsection of the Indian Academy of Neurology as chair and secretary. He regularly presents academic papers at national and international conferences. He has been executive editor of the *Medical Journal Armed Forces India and the Journal of Indian Academy of Geriatrics.*

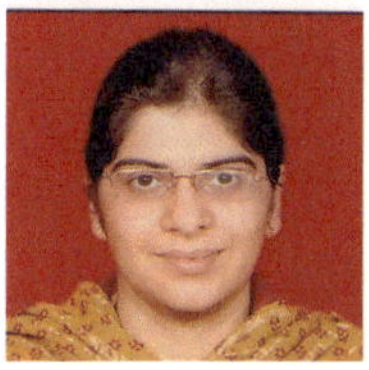

Dr. Kirti Sachdev has been a consultant neurologist at Medipulse Hospital, Jodhpur, India for the last five years. She received her MD with a gold medal from Pt. Ravi Shankar Shukla University Raipur (CG) in 2008 and super specialization DM in neurology from Dr. SN Medical College, Jodhpur in 2017. She has been involved in many published research works in the field of neurology. Her areas of interest are stroke, dementia, and movement disorders. She is a life member of the Indian Academy of Neurology, stroke and movement disorder subsections.

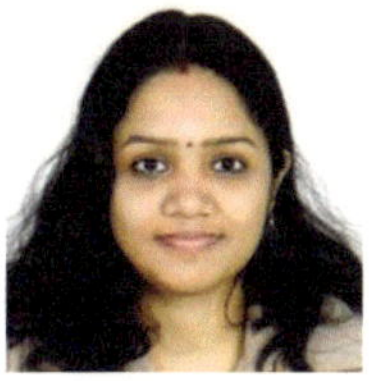

Dr R. Rajeswari is a consultant neurologist at Medipulse Hospital, Jodhpur. She completed her MD in general medicine at Coimbatore Medical College Hospital in 2017 and her DNB in neurology at Sir Gangaram Hospital, New Delhi in 2021. She worked as an academician at the Army College of Medical Sciences, New Delhi from 2017-2018. Her areas of research interest include stroke, epilepsy, multiple sclerosis, and nerve and muscle disorders.

Contents

Preface

Facial nerve palsy is frequently encountered by physicians in outpatient departments. In the post-COVID era, there has been a surge in the number of patients presenting with this common condition. While it is extremely important to identify clinical cues indicating the need for further investigation, a good clinical sense, and knowledge of the causes, can avoid unnecessary investigations and spare patients both cost and anxiety.

This book aims to improve understanding of facial paralysis, its early diagnosis and prompt medical management for physicians, neurologists, postgraduate medical students in medicine and neurology, and physiotherapists. The expression 'time is brain', understood by neurologists and physicians worldwide, acknowledges the importance of early intervention.

In "Medical System to Evaluate the Seventh Cranial Nerve through the Main Facial Mimic Muscles", Martınez-Angeles et al. suggest a novel system for quantifying muscle activity and displaying differential information from both hemifaces.

A multidisciplinary team approach is essential when there is no prospect of further recovery of facial nerve function. Synkinesis and facial spasm are uncommon sequels in partially recovered patients. Mingazova et al., in their article "Comprehensive Rehabilitation of Patients with Facial Expression Asymmetry and Synkinesis with Botulinum Toxin Type A and Monofilament Mesothreads", propose a novel rehabilitation technique that uses botulinum toxin in hypertonic muscles on the healthy side. Facial deformity with impaired function is a sequel in some of the patients.

In their article, "Reanimation of Mouth Corner with Free Gracilis Muscle Flap", Nasir and Cirak successfully employ one session of partial thickness free gracilis muscle flap with innervations from the masseter nerve.

Cheng et al., in "Management of Bell's Palsy with Phototherapy", suggest phototherapy as a safe and promising treatment in conjunction with standard medication. They emphasize that the use of early phototherapy during the acute and subacute stages of the illness is more effective than during the chronic stage.

Dr. Pratap Sanchetee, DM (Neurology)
Consultant Neurologist,
Sanchetee Hospital,
Jodhpur, India

Dr. Kirti Sachdeva, DM (Neurology)
Consultant Neurologist,
MediPulse Hospital,
Jodhpur, India

Dr. R. Rajeshwari, DNB (Neurology)
Consultant Neurologist,
MediPulse Hospital,
Jodhpur, India

Chapter 1

Introductory Chapter: Bell's Palsy

Pratap Sanchetee

1. Introduction

The seventh cranial nerve, commonly known as the facial nerve, is a compound nerve having motor, parasympathetic, and sensory components. Its motor portion innervates muscles for facial movement and expression. In addition, it is involved in taste over the anterior two-third of the tongue. Its parasympathetic component supplies secretomotor fibers to submandibular and sublingual salivary glands and the lacrimal gland. A small twig of this nerve carries sensations from the pinna and the external auditory meatus.

Facial paralysis is a common clinical condition that significantly impacts a patient's quality of life [1]. Seventh cranial nerve paralysis has been categorized as supranuclear if the lesion is above its nucleus in the pons and as intranuclear if the lesion is below the nucleus. This categorization is important from diagnostic, therapeutic, and prognostic points of view and must be made clinically at the initial presentation itself. The peripheral facial nerve palsy, popularly known as Bell's palsy, is an acute disorder of the facial nerve, which produces full or partial loss of voluntary movement on one side of the face. Less common features are loss of taste sensation over the ipsilateral half of the tongue, hyperacusis, tingling or numbness of the cheek/mouth, and ocular pain.

2. Historical perspective

James Douglas (1675–1742) in the eighteenth century gave the description of unilateral facial paralysis. However, Cornelis Stalpart van der Wiel in 1683 first clearly observed and recorded a case that was later described as Bell's palsy. Sir Charles Bell (1774–1842), Scottish surgeon anatomist, and First Professor of Anatomy and Surgery at the Royal College of Surgeons, London, is credited with the first authentic description of the anatomy of the facial nerve and its association with the idiopathic peripheral facial palsy in 1821 [2].

3. Emotional vs. volitional facial paresis

Perhaps the most difficult and poorly understood component of facial palsy is the distinction between voluntary and emotionally driven facial expressions. It must be appreciated that human facial emotional expression is a complex phenomenon resulting from the summation of activity of a large-scale neural network in the cerebral cortex [2]. Gower's description provides an early description of a clinical dissociation between voluntary and emotionally driven facial expressions [3, 4]. Emotional facial paresis results in impaired activation of face muscles with emotion but normal voluntary activation. In contrast, volitional facial paresis such as Bell's palsy results in facial weakness on voluntary effort while emotional movements are preserved [5].

4. Diagnosis

A diagnosis of Bell's palsy is essentially a clinical one and is based on the exclusion of potential other causes of facial weakness. Thorough clinical evaluations suffice in most cases, and they do not require elaborate investigations. Risk factors for Bell's palsy include pregnancy, preeclampsia, obesity, hypertension, diabetes, and upper respiratory ailments. The etiology, prognosis, and degree of facial paralysis are quite variable, and it is not possible to draw a treatment plan which fits to all [1, 6]. Thus, we must exclude other causes of facial palsy in the first instance.

MRI studies are needed on the suspicion of intracranial lesions such as tumors, stroke, and demyelination [7]. The role of electrophysiological tests such as nerve excitability test, maximum stimulation test, electroneuronography, electromyography, etc., though limited in diagnosis, is recommended for assessing regeneration of the nerve and synkinesia.

5. Prognosis

In most instances, patients with Bell's palsy recover completely within approximately 6 months without any treatment [8]. However, 20–30% of patients will have residual facial paresis and disfigurement. Half of such patients (approximately 10–15%) will have moderate-to-severe sequelae such as dysarthria, hemifacial spasm, abnormal lacrimation while eating (crocodile tears), contractures, and synkinesis. In general, children have better outcomes [9]. It has been observed that patients with axonal nerve injury have poorer recovery than those with demyelination. Electrophysiological studies may help us in identifying such subjects.

6. Treatment

To achieve a good cosmetic, and functional recovery, reduction of neuronal damage and prevention of sequel, medical management for Bell's palsy can be categorized into two, i.e., pharmacotherapy and physiotherapy [8]. Surgery is rarely an option for the management of Bell's palsy.

Till recently, corticosteroid was the only drug in our armamentarium to tackle Bell's palsy. Because of their anti-inflammatory mode of action, they can reduce edema and inflammation of the facial nerve. American Academy of Neurology guidelines stated that steroids are highly effective in recovery of facial nerve function in new-onset Bell palsy [10]. Now we have antiviral therapy, which has improved the outcome. Commonly used antiviral agents are acyclovir, famciclovir, and valaciclovir [1]. They can be given concurrently with steroids. The Cochrane review concluded that a small but just significant benefit of combination therapy compared with corticosteroids alone in severe Bell's palsy [11]. To achieve better results, treatment with steroids and antiviral drugs should be initiated at the earliest, preferably within the first week of symptom onset.

Physical therapy, such as exercise, massage, biofeedback, laser treatment, electrostimulation, and thermotherapy, is the backbone of the management of Bell's palsy

[8, 12, 13]. Facial exercises not only hasten recovery during the acute stage but prevent contractures in paralyzed muscles in long term. However, the Cochrane review and other meta-analyses have failed to substantiate tall claims made in many studies. It was concluded that combined physical therapies and steroids plus antiviral drugs may be associated with a better facial function recovery outcome than any single therapy [8, 12].

Kabat rehabilitation, also known as proprioceptive neuromuscular facilitation (PNF), involves the facilitation of the voluntary response of an impaired muscle through the global pattern of an entire muscular section that undergoes resistance [14]. It has shown to be useful to prevent or treat synkinesis. Steroid plus antiviral plus Kabat treatment has shown good facial function recovery [8, 14]. Lately, acupuncture has also been studied as a supplement to other physical therapies. However, these trials are mostly inadequate to draw any conclusions [8, 12, 15]. Hyperbaric oxygen has also been tried to reduce edema over the facial nerve inside the fallopian canal in the temporal bone without any significant clinical recovery [1]. Botulinum toxin can be tried in patients with complications of hemifacial spasm, ipsilateral synkinesis, contralateral hyperkinesis, and facial asymmetry [16].

Most patients with Bell's palsy have reduced blinking ability and protection of eyes from drying, irritation, and injury merit close consideration. Artificial tears or eye ointments or gels, lubricating eye drops, and eye patches are to be used as per the requirement. In severe cases, tarsorrhaphy can also be considered.

7. Surgery

In the past, decompression surgery during the acute stage was tried to relieve the pressure on the facial nerve inside the fallopian canal [8]. However, it has not met with good clinical recovery, and complications such as injury to the facial nerve and permanent hearing loss outweigh the potential benefits. On rare occasions, facial reanimation surgery may be considered in chronic cases for functional and cosmetic benefits.

It can be concluded patients with Bell's palsy should be subjected to combination therapy. Steroid plus antiviral plus Kabat treatment, steroid plus antiviral plus electrical stimulation, and acupuncture plus electrical stimulation have shown promising results in patients with Bell's palsy [8]. However, high-quality trials are needed to recommend any one of them for promising results.

Author details

Pratap Sanchetee
Sanchetee Neurology Research Institute, Jodhpur, India

*Address all correspondence to: pratap.sanchetee@gmail.com

References

[1] Zhao Y, Feng G, Gao Z. Advances in diagnosis and non-surgical treatment of Bell's palsy. The Journal of Otolaryngology. 2015;**10**(1):7-12

[2] Shelley BP. Historical perspectives of facial palsy: Before and after Sir Charles Bell to facial emotional expression. Archives of Medical Health Science. 2013;**1**:85-88

[3] Privatdozentin BW, Rodden FA, Rapp A, Erb M, Grodd W, Ruch W. Humor and smiling: Cortical regions selective for cognitive, affective, and volitional components. Neurology. 2006;**66**:887-889

[4] Gowers WR. A Manual of Diseases of the Nervous System, Vol. 2: Diseases of the Brain and Cranial Nerves; General and Functional Diseases of the Nervous System. London (UK): Forgotten Books; 2019

[5] Hopf HC, Muller-Forell W, Hopf NJ. Localization of emotional and volitional facial paresis. Neurology. 1992;**42**:1918-1923

[6] Kim C, Lelli GJ Jr. Current considerations in the management of facial nerve palsy. Current Opinion in Ophthalmology. 2013;**24**(5):478-483

[7] Sanchetee P. Current trends in stroke rehabilitation. In: Sanchetee P, editor. Ischemic Stroke. London: IntechOpen; 2021

[8] Shi J, Lu D, Chen H, Shu M, Xu Y, Qian J, et al. Efficacy and safety of pharmacological and physical therapies for Bell's palsy: A Bayesian network meta-analysis. Frontiers in Neurology. 2022;**13**:868121

[9] Pavlou E, Gkampeta A, Arampatzi M. Facial nerve palsy in childhood. Brain & Development. 2011;**33**(8):644-650

[10] Gronseth GS, Paduga R. Evidence-based guideline update: Steroids and antivirals for Bell palsy: Report of the Guideline Development Subcommittee of the American Academy of Neurology. Neurology. 2012;**79**(22):2209-2213

[11] Gagyor I, Madhok VB, Daly F, Somasundara D, Sullivan M, Gammie F, et al. Antiviral treatment for Bell's palsy (idiopathic facial paralysis). Cochrane Database of Systematic Reviews. 2015;7:CD001869

[12] Teixeira LJ, Valbuza JS, Prado GF. Physical therapy for Bell's palsy (idiopathic facial paralysis). Cochrane Database of Systematic Reviews. 2011;**12**(12):CD006283

[13] Sanchetee P. Role of yoga and spirituality in stroke rehabilitation. In: Sanchetee P, editor. Ischemic Stroke. London: IntechOpen; 2022

[14] Sharman MJ, Cresswell AG, Riek S. Proprioceptive neuromuscular facilitation stretching: Mechanisms and clinical implications. Sports Medicine (Auckland, NZ). 2006;**36**:929

[15] Chen N, Zhou M, He L, Zhou D, Li N. Acupuncture for Bell's palsy. Cochrane Database of Systematic Reviews. 2010;**2010**(8):CD002914

[16] Cooper L, Lui M, Nduka C. Botulinum toxin treatment for facial palsy: A systematic review. Journal of Plastic, Reconstructive & Aesthetic Surgery. 2017;**70**(6):833-841

Chapter 2

Medical System to Evaluate the Seventh Cranial Nerve through the Main Facial Mimic Muscles

Wendy Liliana Martínez Angeles,
Gregorio Guadalupe-Carbajal Arizaga,
Orfil González-Reynoso and Mario Alberto García-Ramírez

Abstract

Facial palsy is one of the most frequent mononeuropathies expressed in muscular weakness. The condition is produced by lesions in the seventh cranial nerve that causes esthetic, functional, and psychosocial alterations. The disorder has a qualitative diagnosis, and as a consequence, it does hinder the disease timely monitoring. As time is a key factor for the patient's recovery, we developed a system capable to quantify the condition and/or damage in the seventh cranial nerve. It allows us to provide the best treatment available that offers the best response to each patient. To know the seventh cranial nerve state is possible due to the connections between whole muscular system and neurons. The system quantifies the muscles activity and displays the differential information of both hemifaces. Our proposal features a mask in which an array of sensors is placed across the frontal, zygomatic minor, risorio, zygomatic major muscles of each hemiface. The data collected are analyzed and displayed in a user-friendly interface.

Keywords: facial palsy, algorithm, characterization, Bell's palsy, rehabilitation and treatment

1. Introduction

"The facial expressions of human beings fascinate me because they convey both the lowest, most bestial pleasures and the strongest and gentlest emotions of the spirit." This is how Sir Charles Bell described the facial mimic importance [1]. Facial palsy is a disease that reduces the facial symmetry, and as a consequence, it causes functional and esthetic alterations that affect the person mental health as well as the activities they perform on daily basis.

Facial palsy is a disorder that, in most cases, is evaluated qualitatively; therefore, it is essential to find an adequate method to use for diagnosis regardless of the evaluator perception. In this manner, a system capable to quantify the paralyzed hemiface was proposed and developed. Our proposal considers the healthy hemiface as the base control one for the facial palsy and for a bilateral one, the system will use both to evaluate the paralysis degree and to provide an accurate and safer diagnosis in contrast with the nerve conduction diagnosis. Muscular information based on the current status as well as the muscular evolution movement will be gathered by the set of sensors array that would be able to measure the acceleration caused by the muscular movement at each hemiface. As a result of such analysis, it would be possible to deliver an optimal treatment as well as to execute it for each particular case.

2. Facial palsy

Facial palsy is defined as the control loss of the facial muscles due to a dysfunction of the seventh cranial nerve (facial nerve). It can be categorized as complete in the case of the inability to contract the facial muscles voluntarily, hyperacusis, and partial or total taste loss [2–4]. The person who suffers it has a severe disability as the facial nerve is the backbone in facial mimic [4–10].

2.1 Pathology description

The facial nerve has a high-frequency damage rate than any other nerve in the body. It does make peripheral facial palsy the most common cranial mononeuropathy; however, in some cases, when it is not possible to determine or define the cause of origin and only when it is the case, it is designated as Bell's palsy. Although, the origin is attributed as a result of the swelling or facial nerve entrapment in its bony canal within the temporal bone [2, 5–14]; usually, only one side of the face is affected. It might reduce the functionality of both sides. Although, it is uncommon, it is called bilateral facial palsy [1, 2, 4]. Due to the lack of etiology, the treatment of Bell's palsy is deficient in most cases. Fortunately, spontaneous recovery is common [13]. The clinical picture of peripheral facial palsy lies on the lesion localization. Owing to the damage, it inhibits the electrical connections among the facial nerve and the muscles closely related to the affected area. In case that the damage occurs in the nerve conduit that connects the brain to the facial muscles, it is called central facial palsy.

2.2 Facial nerve

The seventh cranial nerve, also known as facial nerve shown in **Figure 1**, originates from the brainstem and travels through the internal auditory and fallopian canals as well as the large parotid. It innervates the orbicularis oris, salivary glands, lacrimal glands, and 23 paired facial muscles via the posterior auricular, temporal, zygomatic, buccal, marginal mandibular, and cervical branches [12].

2.3 Etiology

Facial palsy causes have been encompassed into four possible mechanisms: genetic, due to hereditary factors that have shown to be important. Vascular, where the edema occurs due to insufficient blood supply. Infectious causes. Undetermined etiologies and autoimmune processes. **Table 1** lists the peripheral facial palsy, and **Table 2** lists bilateral facial palsy causes found in the literature [2, 11, 12, 16]. Moreover, viral infections, ischemia, or autoimmune diseases have been postulated as possible pathomechanisms for Bell's palsy [2, 4, 14, 17].

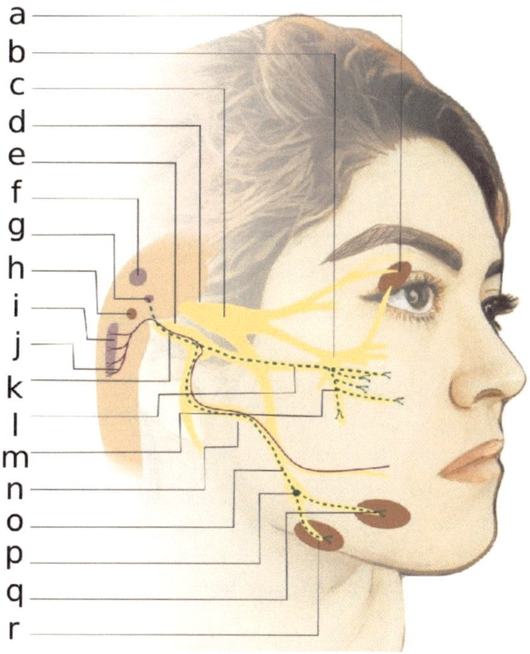

Figure 1.
Schematic diagram that features the facial nerves. The green lines show the parasympathetic fibers. The purple line is the visceral afferent fibers [15]. The labels states for: (a) lacrimal gland, (b) pterygopalatine ganglion, (c) trigeminal ganglion, (d) V n, (e) geniculate ganglion, (f) motor nucleus VI n, (g) superior salivatory nucleus, (h) motor nucleus VII n, (i) fasciculus solitarius, (j) nucleus fasciculus solitarius, (k) VII n, (l) major superficial petrosal nerve, (m) to nasal and palatine glands, (n) chorda tympani, (o) lingual nerve, (p) submandibular gland, (q) sublingual gland, and (r) submandibular gland.

Peripheral facial palsy causes			
Lesions	**Nerve compression**	**Infection, inflammation and virus**	**Others**
			Autism
		SARS-CoV-2	*Asperger
Petrous bone fracture		Influenza	Melkersson-R
Middle ear surgery		Hansen's disease	Metabolic damage
Mastoidectomy		Mastoiditis	
Parotid gland Surgery		Tuberculous meningitis	Histiocytosis
Odotological	Meningioma		Leukemia
surgeries	Cholesteatoma	Nerocysticercosis	Lymphoma
Parotid abscess	Parotid gland tumor	Otitis	Parkinson's
Removal of tumors	Metastasis	Toxocarosis	Preeclampsia
Myasthenia gravis	Meningeosis carcinomatosa	Sarcoidosis	Drugs
Pontine lesions	Facial nerve neuroma	Melkersson-Rosenthal	*Interferon

Peripheral facial palsy causes			
Lesions	**Nerve compression**	**Infection, inflammation and virus**	**Others**
*Tegmental pontine hemorrhage	Osteoporosis	Varicella	*Linezolid
*Ipsilateral pontine		Cryptococcosis	*Others
Infarction		Sarcoidosis	Immune system
*Vascular		Otitis media	diseases
*Tumor		Toxocarosis	*Multiple sclerosis
*Mumps		Meningitis	Diabetes
		Syphilis	*Systemic Lupus
		Immunodeficiency	*Guillain-Barre
		Borreliosis	Miller-Fisher
			Others

Table 1.
Potential causes for peripheral facial nerve palsy [2, 4, 11, 12, 14, 16–21].

Bilateral facial palsy causes			
Lesions	**Nerve compression**	**Infection, inflammation and virus**	**Others**
			Leukemia
		SARS-CoV-2	Drugs
Bulbospinal atrophy fractures		Borreliosis	*Linezolid
Surgeries		Encephalitis	Immune system
Pontine lesions	Cryptococcal meningitis	Hansen's disease	Diseases
*Gliomas hemorrhage		Syphilis	*Diabetes
		Sarcoidosis	*Lupus
		Guillain-Barré	*Guillain-Barre
		Others	*Miller-Fisher
			Others

Table 2.
Potential causes of bilateral facial nerve palsy [2, 22, 23].

2.4 Syntomatology

One of the main tasks that the facial nerve has is to provide motor innervation. As a consequence, when it is damaged, the patients can present decreased facial expression, abnormal muscle tone, syncynesia, hyperacusis, tearing, irritation, dry eyes, inability to blink, loose lips corners, numbness, pain around the ear and temple, temperature variation sensation, altered sense of taste, and flow of saliva out of the mouth [4, 5, 12, 17, 24, 25]. Those symptoms are closely related to the lesion location in the facial nerve [11]. Others are produced due to the facial nerve generating a sensation in one part of the ear. Moreover, the taste is produced at the anterior (two-thirds) of the tongue via the chorda tympani and to the innervation to the lacrimal gland and submandibular one [2, 26].

2.5 Diagnosis

The facial palsy is diagnosed by an abrupt facial expression alteration due to unilateral or bilateral facial weakness of the facial nerve branches. The healthcare professionals take into account the presence of typical symptoms and signs mentioned elsewhere [2, 4]. Although, Bell's palsy diagnosis is reserved to be used when whole set of peripheral facial palsy causes are excluded. Nevertheless, Bell's palsy can coexist with the diseases that cause peripheral facial palsy [2]. In some cases, blood chemistries, cerebrospinal fluid analysis, mastoids, and crane X-rays, magnetic resonance imaging, or nerve conduction studies for facial nerve prognosis [2]. In contrast, therapeutic functional evaluation includes patient history, initial photographs or video recording of facial movements, electromyographic readings, observations of muscle tone, movement, and synsynesias [5, 12, 27].

Additionally, the weakness progression is evaluated by reviewing old photographs in order to compare it with the current status. The damage degree can also be assessed by the conduction of the facial nerve. A nerve conduction study measures the potential action, amplitude, and latencies through the facial nerve (**Table 3**). The study can identify nerve damage, as an example, the damage degree can also be assessed by nerve conduction of the facial nerve. Decreased muscle-action potentials suggest axon degeneration while increased latency suggests nerve demyelination [2, 28]. Along the test, several electrodes are inserted into the facial muscles. The muscles used to fix the electrodes are the orbicularis oculi or the oblicularis oris, mentalis, messetere, and temporalis. Two electrodes are needed for each muscle. The first electrode sends an electrical stimulation, and the other one is used as an electrical impulse receptor. The received signal is used to calculate the nerve conduction velocity [29]. However, prospective analyses are needed to assess the relevance of nerve conduction studies [27].

Usually, electromyography is often performed at the same time. The study measures the muscular electrical activity. It shares the same methodology as the nerve conduction study. The main difference lies in the electrodes distribution. In here, it used superficial electrodes while in the nerve conduction study, the electrodes are invasive. Both studies are searching the damage location in the facial nerve or in the muscles innervated by it [29].

In addition, magnetic resonance imaging is used to detect lesions in the facial nerve [30]. Magnetic resonance imaging or MRI is a technique that uses the magnetic field to generate images of the human body. MRI assesses the underlying disease. In patients with facial palsy, the MRI is used to measure facial muscle volumes by monitoring the decease development [31]. Other authors concluded that contrast enhancement of the paralytic nerve can be indicative of a nerve inflammation. Furthermore, through the MRI image, it is possible to estimate the recovery [30]. Moreover, older facial nerve studies have shown that abnormalities displayed by the MRI were not conclusive to diagnose Bell's palsy [32]. Nevertheless, in 2000, according to the authors, it was find an abnormal MRI in bilateral Bell's palsy [33].

Bilateral facial palsy causes		
Bulbospinal atrophy	Pontine gliomas	Mononucleosis
Borreliosis	Pontine hemorrhage	Sífilis
Diabetes	Infections	Sarcoidosis
Pregnancy	Leprosy	Guillain-Barré
Encephalitis	Leukemia	Miller-Fisher
Hansen's disease	Systemic lupus erythematosus	Moebius
Fractures	Cryptococcal meningitis	Linezolid therapy

Table 3.
Potential causes of bilateral facial nerve palsy [2, 22, 23].

2.6 Palsy grade analysis

Measurement scales to clinically assess facial palsy severity and population studies differ among researchers [34]. In order to standardize the paralysis classification, several scales have been developed such as the Sunderland, Sunnybrook, the Yanagihara classification system, and the most widely used, the House-Brackmann system shown in **Table 4** [2, 4, 12, 34–39]. The most used systems rely on the resting symmetry assessment, facial-muscles excursion degree, and triggered synkinesis by performing voluntary specific movements [2, 40].

The palsy-degrees qualitative descriptions make a clinical evaluation quite complicated. Furthermore, a misunderstood etiology makes the prognosis unpredictable. It also provokes a sluggish pathological process that as a consequence affects the patient recovery [13].

2.7 Rehabilitation

Rehabilitation focuses on regaining voluntary muscle contraction, improving movement quality, synkinesis control, enhancing symmetry, and increasing the percentage of facial functionality. It is important to achieve a fast recovery to reach a complete restoration of muscle function. Literature shows that the faster the recovery, the less sequelae will be [5, 11, 12, 14, 41]. In addition, the recovery time is key between the second and the fourth week. Thence, to find the most suitable treatment for each patient in the shortest time is essential. A facial palsy poorly treated might cause functional difficulties that decrease the patient's ability to communicate. Psychological help is also essential as it also generates cosmetic deformities that provide serious social stigma to the person who suffers it [2, 5, 12, 14].

Peripheral facial palsy rehabilitation is based on treating the underlying disorder. However, for Bell's palsy case (unknown etiology), the treatment has been controversial due to the lack of scientific evidence. Moreover, it is possible that the diseases listed as the triggers for facial palsy are also present in patients with paresis without being the cause for Bell's palsy [2, 11, 42]. On the other hand, anti-inflammatories and antivirals have shown a major recovery index in patients with Bell's palsy [14, 43, 44].

Balliet in 1982 focused on the study of facial mimic. He proposed a set of key therapeutic exercises to activate muscles or to evoke localized movements [27, 45]. In

Grade	HBS	Y system (%)
Normal, symmetric functions in all areas.	I	40
Mild weakness on close inspection, complete closure of eyes with minimal effort, asymmetrical weakness of smile with maximal effort, weak synkinesis, no contractures or spasms.	II	32–38
Obvious but not disfiguring weakness of the face, inability to raise the eyebrow, full and forceful eye closures, asymmetric movement of the mouth with maximal effort, obvious but not disfiguring synkinesis, mass movement or twitching.	III	24–30
Obvious disfigurement due to weakness, inability to raise the eyebrows, incomplete closure of the eyes, asymmetry of the mouth with maximum effort, severe synkinesis, mass movements, spasms.	IV	16–22
Barely perceptible movement, incomplete closure of eyes, weak movement at the corner of the mouth, synkinesis, contracture, spasms usually absent.	V	8–14
No movement, low muscle tone, no synkinesis, contracture and spasms.	VI	0–6

Table 4.
House-Brackmann (HBS) and Yanagihara classification systems to rate the severity of facial nerve palsy by evaluating the forehead motility, eyes, nose, and mouth [2, 37].

addition, in order to increase the operative facial movements, inhibit abnormal movements, maintain trophism, and provide tactile stimulation, techniques such as neuromuscular retraining, isolated exercises, stimulation of sensory modulation, acupuncture, application butyllium toxin, electrical stimulation, surgery, massage, and vibratory therapy are highly used [4, 5, 12]. However, further research is needed regarding specific indications, duration of rehabilitation and potential recovery [2, 5, 12, 14].

2.8 Prevalence

The facial palsy incidence is estimated between 11 and 40 cases per 100,000 inhabitants annually [2, 4, 11, 14, 15]. The peak incidence occurs between 15 and 45 years. However, one in 60 people will experience it in their lifetime [15]. The prevalence of bilateral facial palsy spans from 0.3 to 2%, it increases in pregnant women, diabetic patients, respiratory diseases, influenza or has attended an extraction of a tooth root. It is not common in children under 2 years of age [2, 17].

2.9 Prognosis

The people prognosis with paresis depends on two main factors, the paralysis degree, and the individual age. The younger the patient, the better the prognosis. When a facial palsy is incomplete, over 94% of patients recover their face functionality [6, 27, 46–49]. In a facial palsy, if recovery does not occur within the first 6 months, the long-term clinical picture includes speech distortion, difficulty to eat, syncynesia, atrophy, soft tissue adherence, and muscle lengthening [12]. Some patients also mentioned otalgia or mild retroarticular pain. When the patients present those sequels, their life quality decreases drastically causing impediments in their work and social life [14]. By receiving therapy, the rate of facial palsy recovery may improve after 1 year, in contrast to those who did not receive any treatment [2, 4, 26, 27, 50].

3. COVID-related facial palsy

The SARS-CoV-2 (COVID-19) infection pandemic has been a major public health issue worldwide. Recent studies have shown that it has an effect on other pathologies such as neurological syndromes [21, 51, 52]. COVID-19 as well as facial palsy disrupts the daily life of our society. Those diseases provoke anguish to those who suffer it due to possible functional and esthetic sequels [21, 51]. Literature has suggested a possible link between COVID-19 and facial palsy, the coronavirus neurotropic nature [21]. The COVID-19 ability to infect different cell types is determined by the ACE2 receptors. The ACE2 inhibitors are located at the endothelial cells of the blood-brain barrier. The binding between ACE2 and COVID-19 allows it to enter the central nervous system [52, 52, 55], even facial palsy has been proposed as the first and only COVID-19 symptom [54, 56].

The COVID-19 incidence has increased along the pandemic development, and some studies focus on the vaccine trial as facial palsy cause [21]. Although, other authors do not find significant differences in the incidence of facial palsy [57], the incidence in pregnant women increases due to the physiological pregnancy stress. This is why they could be more susceptible to neurotropic invasion by the virus [52]. It has been reported an unusual amount of children, a cluster of six, that features facial palsy between March 23 and April 26, 2020 [58]. Despite the low incidence, the bilateral facial palsy case was reported as an asymptomatic COVID-19 [59]. Later, other bilateral facial palsy studies related to COVID-19 were presented [60, 61].

Authors hypothesize in their works that Bell's palsy may be a neuro-COVID-19 manifestation. Nevertheless, a few authors have claimed that there is not enough evidence to establish a clear cause between the two conditions [21, 52, 56, 57]. Other researchers compile the online databases about COVID-19 and facial palsy, and they concluded that COVID-19 increases the number of neurological deceases and pointed out that SARS-CoV-2 infection may be an underlying etiology in patients with COVID-19, and facial palsy can be the first COVID-19 manifestation [62, 63].

4. Our system proposal

In order to support and help patients that suffer facial palsy as well as the professionals who treat them, a system to analyze the illness was developed. Our proposal features two modules: WaLi that is an electronic device that it is responsible for data aqcuisition and a graphical user-friendly interface called WaL that displays the processed data.

WaLi is a system that features a set of sensors distributed across the face in which are localized the muscles controlled by the seventh nerve. **Figure 1** shows a schematic image that features the seventh cranial nerve following an axial symmetry. At each point shown in **Figure 2(a)**, a set of sensors will be distributed on the same spot to measure each muscle in a differential way.

In order to measure the movement provided by the muscles, eight inertial measurement units that features six freedom degrees were used. The sensors were placed at the frontal, zygomaticus minor, zygomaticus major, risorius, and the pairs by following an axial symmetry. The data generated by the muscles and transmitted to the sensors are sent through several data busses. Although, WaLi (**Figure 3**) is a physical array of electronics devices, it needs software to execute a set of algorithms on the acquired data. The backbone of the software is the acquisition algorithm that is

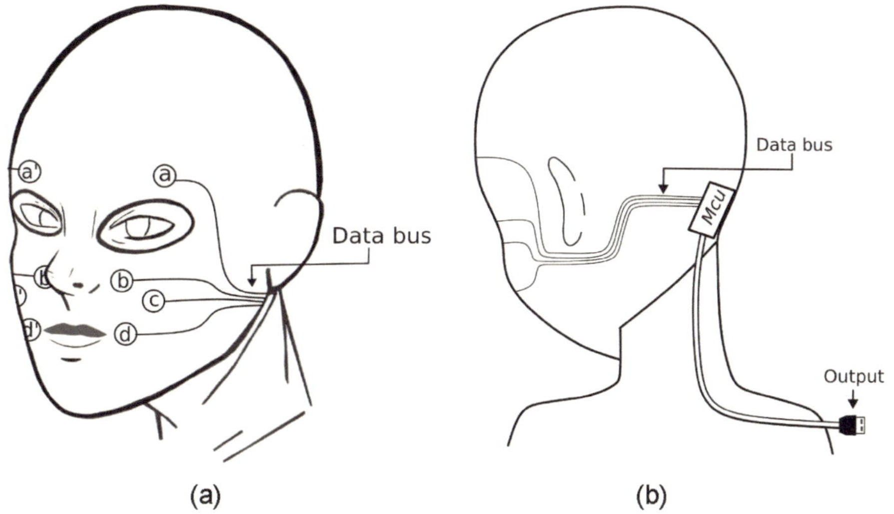

Figure 2.
Schematic diagram that features hardware system. (a) The circles show the sensor location on the most representative muscles of the facial mimic (frontal, minor zygomatic, risorio, and the major zygomatic) and (b) the data bus that links the sensors to the MCU at the rear.

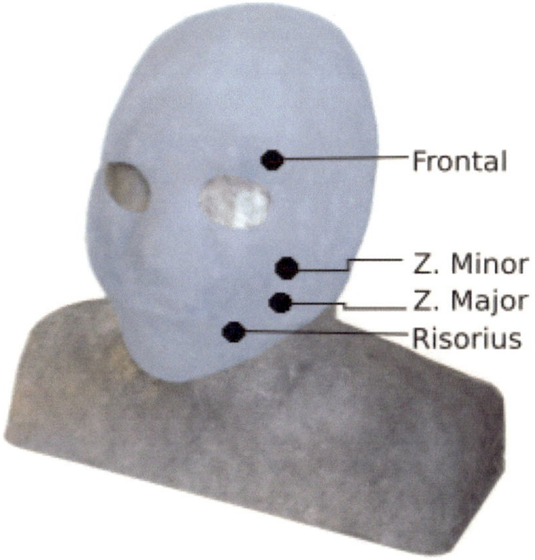

Figure 3.
Schematic diagram that shows the sensors distribution across the both hemifaces over the key muscles.

responsible to gather the data and sending it to the serial port by using a serial communication protocol.

The facial symmetry is the key principle in which the system is based. This is why, the backbone of the entire system focuses on the position at which each sensor is located across the face. In order to keep the position sharp for each sensor, a mask was developed through the fabrication of positive and negative mold. Once the sensors were in place on the key spots, the data busses were positioned in order to not interfere with the facial mimic. Once fixed, the negative mold was used to finish the mask to keep the whole set of arrays in place.

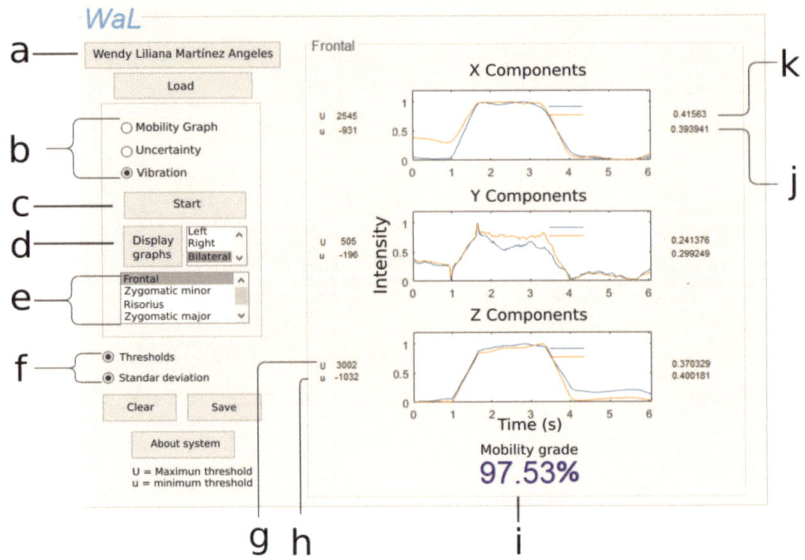

Figure 4.
Schematic diagram that shows WaL, the user-friendly interface. In here, it shows the mobility graphs of the frontal muscle in a healthy person. The left side exhibits a set of menus that the user can utilize. The options to manipulate are: (a) patient information; (b) study type; (c) start study; (d) display graphs and hemiface; (e) muscle to show; (f) thresholds and standard deviation; (g) maximum threshold; (h) minimum threshold, (i) mobility degree; (k) and (j) standard deviation of left and right hemiface, respectively.

WaL: It is defined as a user-friendly interface that receives, analyzes, and displays the information obtained from the muscles chosen by the user. **Figure 4** shows a schematic diagram that displays the interface featuring the mobility behavior of a healthy person.

For the development of WaL, a set of algorithms based on numerical analyses were used. The interface established a serial communication between WaLi and WaL in order to collect the data from the serial port. The data are sent through a serial port as a vector. WaL stores and transforms the vector into a matrix. The columns are classified as a function of the hemiface, muscle name, and the plane in which the movement was performed (x, y, and z). Then, the signal is preprocessed to be analyzed later. No human is symmetrical; hereby, at the interface, the user selects the healthy hemiface. The option selected by the user will be considered by the algorithm as a reference. The robustness of the system allows to be used by anyone due to the user-friendly interface.

Another feature that WaL has is the postprocessing feature. A set of statistical analyses can be performed on WaL such as standard deviation, mean, and correlation coefficient. Furthermore, another measurement unit was proposed [64]. The mobility degree (gM) expressed as a percentage of the weakened hemiface as function of the healthy counterpart is obtained by using the following equation:

$$gM = \frac{100 \times \left(a_{2f} - a_{2i}\right)}{a_f - a_i} \tag{1}$$

where a_{2i}: initial component of the weakened hemiface; a_{2f}: final component in x, y or z of the weakened hemiface; a_i: initial component of the healthy hemiface; a_f: final component of the healthy hemiface.

Moreover, WaL is capable to analyze and display the state and the information that each sensor has as well as auto-calibration, patient information, and the option to safe the analysis.

5. Statistical and behavioral analysis

In order to show the effectiveness of the system, a study on muscular trajectory was performed in 18 patients for male and female genders on an age span of 22 and 24 years. Fifteen of the patients were healthy, and three presented peripheral facial palsy. The protocol to analyze the group of patients was as follows: the test subject sat in a chair with a straight back making sure that he/she was comfortable. Once the test subject was in place, he/she put on the mask and adjusted it so that the sensors were on the corresponding muscle. Immediately WaL started to record. The person contracted the muscles to be studied as intensely as possible for a couple of seconds and immediately relaxed them.

The results found from healthy people were used for calibration purposes. The ill individual results corroborate that our system is capable to quantify the muscle movement controlled by the seventh cranial nerve. The system is calibrated to take 12,000 samples of the muscular trajectory in 6.06 seconds, with this information, the standard deviation and the mean for each component are obtained. The correlation among components of the same muscle such as the thresholds that state the point of major and minor displacement, the asymmetry facial, and muscle correlation is expressed as a percentage. The data that the system collected when conducting the study on the 15 healthy people and three people with facial paralysis were used as a reference to establish the thresholds that indicate the state of the user's facial muscles. The purpose of the system is to provide a tool that contributes with information for an accurate diagnosis. The collected data can reduce the time to find the ideal treatment for the patients. The data measured by the system are graphed and normalized in order to standardize the signal and thus, compare the reaction speed and intensity of the movement of each hemiface.

5.1 Healthy person muscular trajectory

The central trajectory measurements that appear in **Figure 5** correspond to a healthy 24-year-old woman, weighing 70 kg and 1.74 m tall. The frontal muscle trajectory shown in **Figure 5I** has a correlation percentage for all the components of 95.54%, zygomaticus minor (**Figure 5II**) has a correlation of 94.23%, risorio (**Figure 5II**) of 96.42% and for zygomaticus major (**Figure 5IV**) it is 92.61%. Although the study was applied to a healthy person. The asymmetry of the face of this particular person is accentuated in the zygomaticus minor muscle. Therefore, it can be affirmed that the muscular response is attenuated by 7.39%.

5.2 Facial paralysis muscular trajectory

The person with facial paralysis is shown in **Figure 6**. It is observed that the similarity of the signals decreases in all the muscles. By having a correlation percentage of 77.14% for the frontal muscle, 73.30% for the zygomatic minor, 84.60% for the risorius, and 5.48% for the zygomaticus major.

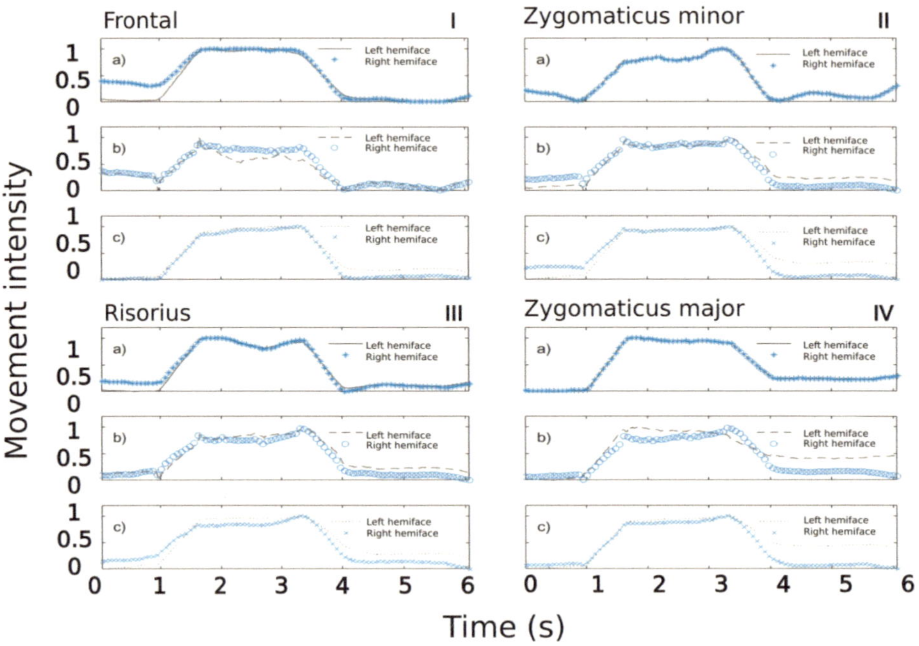

Figure 5.
Set of experimental results that shows the muscle movement intensity in a healthy person where the frontal (I), zigomaticus minor (II), risorius (III), and zigomaticus major (IV) are shown. The signals are normalized and plotted against time (a) shows the "x" components of the muscle trajectory, (b) the "y" components, and (c) shows present the components in "z."

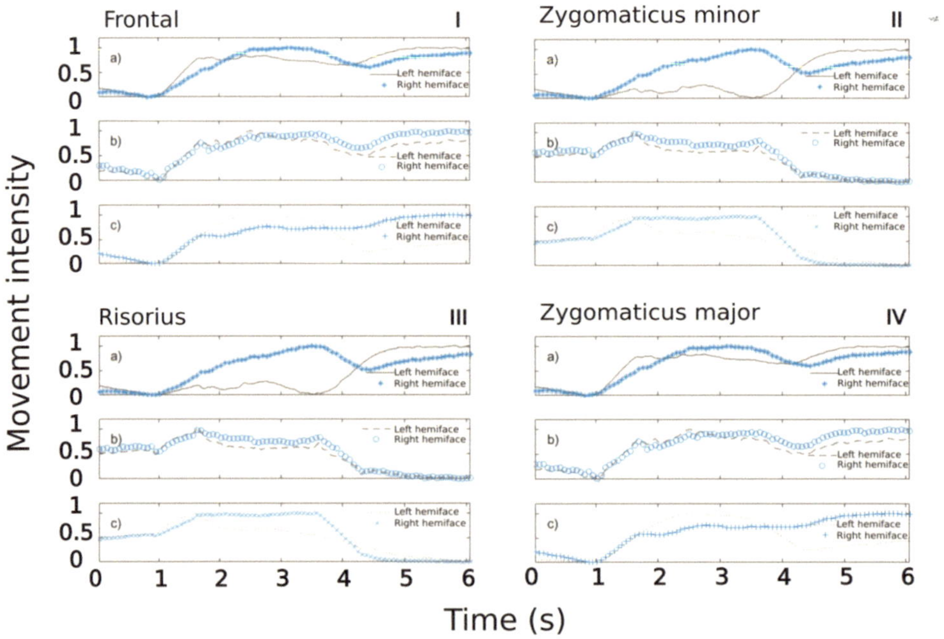

Figure 6.
Set of measured results that feature the intensity of frontal (I), zigomaticus minor (II), risorius (III), and zigomaticus major (IV) muscles movement in a person with facial paralysis. The signals were normalized and are plotted against time where (a), (b), and (c) are the x, y, and z components, respectively.

The signals belong to the injured hemiface that reached the maximum point of contraction starting from the minimum state in a longer time with respect to the healthy counterpart. In most cases, the signals are function of the healthy side of the face by reaching the highest intensity in approximately 1 s while the signals from the paralyzed side take twice as long.

6. Muscle trajectory analysis

In order to show the trajectory analysis, a set of box plots were used to graphically represent the scatter, symmetry, and outliers found in the muscle trajectory signal. On the graph of the healthy person (**Figure** 7), it can be seen that the upper quartile is larger than the lower one. In addition, the mean values of both sides are closer to last mentioned.

The patient that presents facial palsy (**Figure 8**), it is observed that the interquartile distribution of the injured half-face with respect to the healthy half-face is irregular. It does imply that those are not close to any particular quartile. In addition, outliers are presented in the diagram between the lower quartile and the minimum threshold; likewise, the distance between the outer quartiles and the thresholds is greater compared with the diagrams in **Figure** 7.

The outliers denoted by "+" signs outside the quartiles are neither present in the healthy person (**Figure** 7) nor in the healthy person half-face with paralysis box plot (**Figure 8a**). As the study results show, WaL is effective in quantifying the trajectory of the frontalis, zygomaticus minor, risorius, and zygomaticus major muscles. The data obtained from the tests performed on 15 healthy persons and three with facial

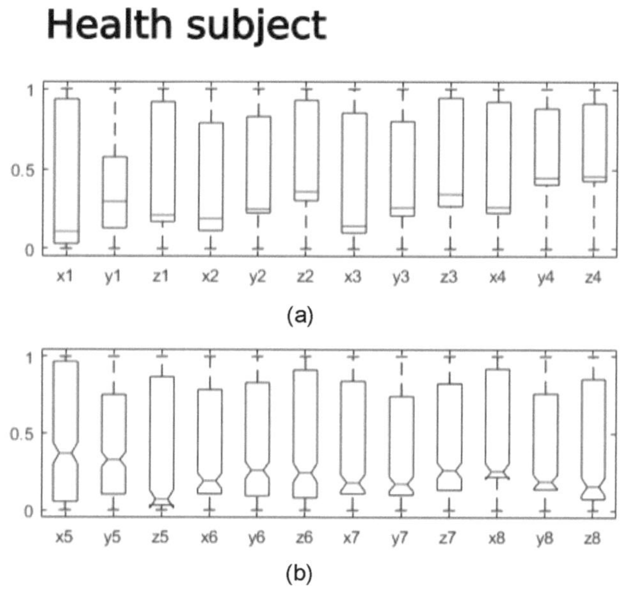

Figure 7.
Muscular trajectory box diagrams in normal state. The names along the x-axis represent the sensor number. (a) Represents the left hemiface side with sensors 1–4 and (b) the right hemiface side with sensors 5–8. Notches were added in the diagrams of the healthy hemiface for purposes of distinction.

paralysis suggest that the facial correlation percentage of a healthy person is in a span between 89.57% and 97.87%, with a deviation standard between 0.34822 and 0.3433.

Due to the fact that having a healthy face does not guarantee having a symmetrical face, the system does a precalibration, by showing an error coefficient in order to express the asymmetry. Under the assumption that all faces are asymmetric, the facial muscles are normal when the error coefficient is below 10.43%.

According to the graphs generated by the system (**Figure 5**), when one side of the face is in a normal state, the average response speed from the point of largest relaxation to the point of largest contraction is 2.49 seconds while for the injured hemifaces, it was 3.52 seconds. Furthermore, it was observed in the experimental data that when the correlation is high, the data dispersion marked by the standard deviation increases.

From the analyses shown in **Figures** 7 and **8**, it is observed that if the contraction muscle time is larger than the relaxation time, the length of the upper quartiles increase; on the other hand, it decreases if the contraction is lower, so it can be stated that the length of the quartiles depends on the muscle contraction as well as the mean. Although the possibility of anomalous values + that appear in the box plots of normalized signals from healthy half-faces is not ruled out, in the 18 studies on which this research is based, outliers were only present in the normalized paralyzed hemifaces.

The person whose results are shown in **Figure 6** was diagnosed with peripheral facial paralysis. It shows weakness on the left side of the face, which was confirmed by the system with an average standard deviation of 0.32232 and a facial correlation coefficient of 72.63%. A value that is outside of the range previously established for healthy people, which means that the electrical potentials presented the muscles of the left side of the face were attenuated by 27.37% due to the paralysis, by making it impossible for the person to perform a symmetrical contraction affecting their muscular excursion.

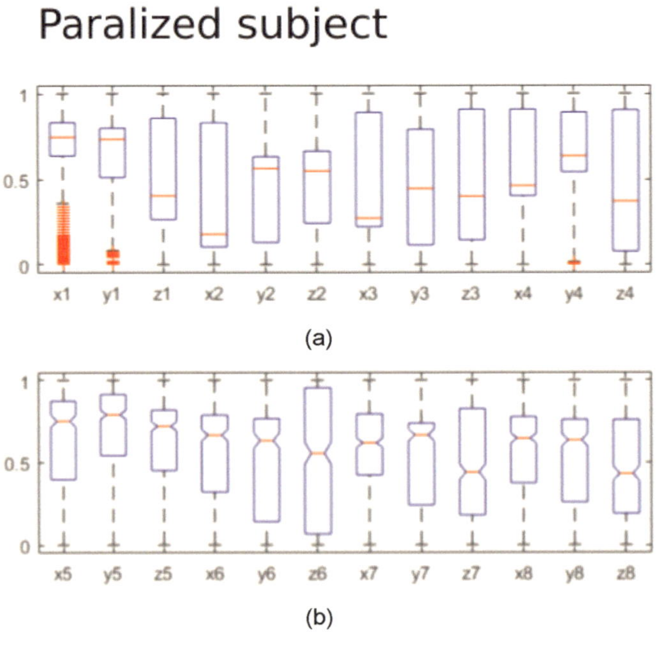

Figure 8.
*Muscle trajectory box plots, those represent a person with facial palsy. (a) Shows the components of the left hemiface side muscles on the left hemiface side and (b) the right hemiface side. In addition, both hemifaces display an odd behavior (a) and (b), in contrast with a healthy person shown elsewhere (**Figure 7**).*

7. Conclusions

A full system to quantify the degree of facial palsy that will help to know the degree of muscle re–education improvement or not with the help of therapy was proposed and fabricated. By broadening the panorama of possible disease causes and keeping a timely record. An important point in performing the study with WaLi and WaL system is the placement of the mask, as the sensors are not located on the muscle to which they have been assigned, the result will be affected. By accentuating the degree of error of the system in the axis from which it was erroneously offset with respect to the point of interest.

For a face to be classified as healthy, it must have a high correlation, which means that the movement of both sides is very similar in intensity and time. According to the results provided by the system, healthy faces have a shorter response time between the largest relaxation point to the longest contraction that causes the difference between the mean of the signal and the data by increasing the standard deviation. So, it can be concluded that the greater the deviation, the correlation coefficient, and the arithmetic mean, the greater the symmetry of the face and the smaller the difference in reaction time.

Acknowledgements

We express our gratitude to the Mexican National Council of Science and Technology (CONACYT) for their support under the Scholarship 1023006 and the Research Project 319712 as well as the Chemistry & Electronics Department and the Methabolic and Bioinformatic Lab of University of Guadalajara.

Conflict of interest

The authors declare no conflict of interest.

Author details

Wendy Liliana Martínez Angeles[1†], Gregorio Guadalupe-Carbajal Arizaga[1†], Orfil González-Reynoso[1†] and Mario Alberto García-Ramírez[1,2*†]

1 Research Centre for Applied Science and Engineering (CUCEI), Universidad de Guadalajara, Guadalajara, Mexico

2 Research Centre for Translational Medicine (CiMeT), Guadalajara, Mexico

*Address all correspondence to: mario.garcia@academicos.udg.mx

† These authors contributed equally.

References

[1] Bell C. The nervous system of the human body. Archives of Neurology. 1969;**21**(6):662-666

[2] Finsterer J. Management of peripheral facial nerve palsy. European Archives of Oto-Rhino-Laryngology. 2008;**265**(7): 743-752

[3] Sepulveda JJO, Amor JJO. Ondine's curse during pregnancy. Journal of Neurology, Neurosurgery & Psychiatry. 2005;**76**(2):294-294

[4] Palacio CAC, Galarza FAM. Cutaneous sensibility changes in Bell's palsy patients. Otolaryngology—Head and Neck Surgery (United States). 2017; **156**(5):828-833

[5] Dalla Toffola E et al. Usefulness of bfb/emg in facial palsy rehabilitation. Disability and Rehabilitation. 2005; **27**(14):809-815

[6] Peitersen E. Bell's palsy: The spontaneous course of 2,500 peripheral facial nerve palsies of different etiologies. Acta Oto-Laryngologica. Supplementum. 2002;**549**:4-30

[7] Peitersen E. Natural history of bell's palsy. Acta Oto-Laryngologica. 1992;**112** (sup492):122-124

[8] Leibowitz U. Epidemic incidence of bell's palsy. Brain. 1969;**92**(1):109-114

[9] May M, Hardin WB. Facial palsy: Interpretation of neurologic findings. The Laryngoscope. 1978;**88**(8): 1352-1362

[10] Novak CB et al. Facial sensibility in patients with unilateral facial nerve paresis. Otolaryngology-Head and Neck Surgery. 1993;**109**(3):506-513

[11] Roob G et al. Peripheral facial palsy: Etiology, diagnosis and treatment. European Neurology. 1999;**41**(1):3-9

[12] Cronin GW, Steenerson RL. The effectiveness of neuromuscular facial retraining combined with electromyography in facial paralysis rehabilitation. Otolaryngology—Head and Neck Surgery. 2003;**128**(4):534-538

[13] Galal S et al. New trends in management of facial nerve paralysis facial. Biolife. 2015;**3**(3):629-638

[14] Hultcrantz M. Rehabilitation of bells' palsy from a multi-team perspective. Acta Oto-Laryngologica. 2016;**136**(4): 363-367

[15] Kasper D, Anthony F, Stephen H, Dan L, Jameson J, Joseph L. Harrison's principles of internal medicine, 19e. Vol. 1, no. 2. New York, NY, USA: Mcgraw-Hill; 2015

[16] Williamson IG, Whelan TR. The clinical problem of bell's palsy: Is treatment with steroids effective? The British Journal of General Practice. 1996; **46**(413):743-747

[17] Slavkin HC. The significance of a human smile: Observations on bell's palsy. The Journal of the American Dental Association. 1999;**130**(2):269-272

[18] Garro A, Nigrovic LE. Managing peripheral facial palsy. Annals of Emergency Medicine. 2018;**71**(5):618-624

[19] Tello M, Gutierrez E, Béjar V, Galarza C, Ramos W, Ortega-Loayza AG. Cryptococcosis. Revista Médica de Risaralda. 2013;**19**(2):147-153

[20] Nachtsheim L, Wittersheim M, Kreissl S, Klussmann JP, Grosheva M.

Facial nerve paralysis caused by a t-cell lymphoma. Clinical Case Reports. 2020; **8**(12):2965

[21] Codeluppi L, Venturelli F, Rossi J, Fasano A, Toschi G, Pacillo F, et al. Facial palsy during the covid-19 pandemic. Brain and Behavior. 2021;**11**(1):e01939

[22] Jeong SM, Park JH, In Lee J, Nam KE, Lee JS, Kim JH. Progressive bilateral facial palsy as a manifestation of granulomatosis with polyangiitis: A case report. Annals of Rehabilitation Medicine. 2016;**40**(4):734-740

[23] Pothiawala S, Lateef F. Bilateral facial nerve palsy: A diagnostic dilemma. Case Reports in Emergency Medicine. Hindawi Publishing Corporation. 2012; **2012**:1-3. Article ID 458371. DOI: 10.1155/2012/458371

[24] Çelik M, Hulki F, Çetin V. The development of synkinesis after facial nerve paralysis. European Neurology. 2000;**43**(3):147-151

[25] Kimura J et al. Electrophysiologic analysis of aberrant regeneration after facial nerve paralysis. Neurology. 1975; **25**(10):989-989

[26] Atzema C, Goldman RD. Should we use steroids to treat children with bell's palsy? Canadian Family Physician. 2006; **52**(3):313-314

[27] Holland NJ et al. Recent developments in bell's palsy. BMJ. 2004; **329**(7465):553-557

[28] Kimura J. Electrodiagnosis of the cranial nerves. Acta Neurologica Taiwanica. 2006;**15**(1):2

[29] Harner SG, Daube JR, Beatty CW, Ebersold MJ. Intraoperative monitoring of the facial nerve. The Laryngoscope. 1988;**98**(2):209-212

[30] Yetiser S, Kazkayas M, Altınok D, Karadeniz Y. Magnetic resonance imaging of the intratemporal facial nerve in idiopathic peripheral facial palsy. Clinical Imaging. 2003;**27**(2):77-81

[31] Volk GF, Karamyan I, Klingner CM, Reichenbach JR, Guntinas-Lichius O. Quantitative magnetic resonance imaging volumetry of facial muscles in healthy patients with facial palsy. Plastic and Reconstructive Surgery Global Open. 2014;**2**(6):1-9

[32] Murphy TP, David CT. Magnetic resonance imaging of the facial nerve during Bell's palsy. Otolaryngology Head and Neck Surgery 1991;**105**(5): 667-674

[33] Shaikh ZA, Bakshi R, Wasay M, Dai A, Gosy E. Magnetic resonance imaging findings in bilateral bell's palsy. Journal of Neuroimaging. 2000;**10**(4):223-225

[34] van Veen MM et al. Association of regional facial dysfunction with facial palsy–related quality of life. JAMA Facial Plastic Surgery. 2019;**21**(1):32-37

[35] Kanerva M et al. Sunnybrook and house-brackmann facial grading systems: Intrarater repeatability and interrater agreement. Otolaryngology—Head and Neck Surgery. 2006;**135**(6): 865-871

[36] Berg T et al. The effect of study design and analysis methods on recovery rates in bell's palsy. The Laryngoscope. 2009;**119**(10):2046-2050

[37] Samsudin WS, Sundaraj K. Evaluation and grading systems of facial paralysis for facial rehabilitation. Journal of Physical Therapy Science. 2013;**25**(4): 515-519

[38] Ahrens A et al. Rapid simultaneous comparison system for subjective

grading scales grading scales for facial paralysis. The American Journal of Otology. 1999;**20**(5):667-671

[39] Sunderland S. Nerve and Nerve Injuries Edinburgh. London: Livingstone; 1968

[40] Ross BG et al. Development of a sensitive clinical facial grading system. Otolaryngology—Head and Neck Surgery. 1996;**114**(3):380-386

[41] Devriese PP. Rehabilitation of facial expression ("mime therapy"). In: The Facial Nerve. Berlin, Heidelberg: Springer; 1994. pp. 42-43

[42] Türk-Börü U et al. The efficacy of steroids in idiopathic facial nerve paralysis: An open, randomized, prospective controlled study. Kulak burun bogaz ihtisas dergisi: KBB = Journal of Ear, Nose, and Throat. 2005;**14**(3–4):62-66

[43] Ferreira M et al. Physical therapy with drug treatment in bell palsy: A focused review. American Journal of Physical Medicine & Rehabilitation. 2015;**94**(4):331-340

[44] Watson, GJ, Glover S, Allen S, Irving RM. Outcome of facial physiotherapy in patients with prolonged idiopathic facial palsy. The Journal of Laryngology & Otology 2015;**129**(4):348-352

[45] Balliet R et al. Facial paralysis rehabilitation: Retraining selective muscle control. International Rehabilitation Medicine. 1982;**4**(2):67-74

[46] Kasse C et al. The value of prognostic clinical data in bell's palsy. Revista Brasileira de Otorrinolaringologia. 2005; **71**(4):454-458

[47] Ünüvar E et al. Corticosteroid treatment of childhood bell's palsy. Pediatric Neurology. 1999;**21**(5):814-816

[48] Devriese PP et al. Incidence, prognosis and recovery of bell's palsy a survey of about 1000 patients (1974–1983). Clinical Otolaryngology & Allied Sciences. 1990;**15**(1):15-27

[49] Adour KK, Wingerd J. Idiopathic facial paralysis (bell's palsy): Factors affecting severity and outcome in 446 patients. Neurology. 1974;**24**(12): 1112-1112

[50] Sittel C et al. Bell's palsy: A 10-year experience with antiphlogistic-rheologic infusion therapy. Otology & Neurotology. 2000;**21**(3):425-432

[51] Lima MA, Silva MTT, Soares CN, Coutinho R, Oliveira HS, Afonso L, et al. Peripheral facial nerve palsy associated with covid-19. Journal of Neurovirology. 2020;**26**(6):941-944

[52] Kumar V, Narayanan P, Shetty S, Mohammed AP. Lower motor neuron facial palsy in a postnatal mother with covid-19. BMJ Case Reports CP. 2021; **14**(3):e240267

[53] Hasibi M, Ahadi MS, Abdollahi H, Jafari M. Protracted covid-19 during treatment of facial palsy. Case Reports in Neurological Medicine. 2021:**2021**:1-3

[54] Islamoglu Y, Celik B, Kiris M. Facial paralysis as the only symptom of covid-19: A prospective study. American Journal of Otolaryngology. 2021;**42**(4): 102956

[55] Mohanan VV, Gayathri K. Viral and host cellular factors used by neurotropic viruses. In The Molecular Immunology of Neurological Diseases. Academic Press; 2021. pp. 75-83

[56] Figueiredo R, Falcão V, Pinto MJ, Ramalho C. Peripheral facial paralysis as presenting symptom of covid-19 in a

pregnant woman. BMJ Case Reports CP. 2020;**13**(8):e237146

[57] Martin-Villares C, Alba JR, Gonzalez-Gimeno MJ. Data from 235 cases of bell's palsy during covid-19 pandemic: Were there clusters of facial palsy? Neuroepidemiology. 2021;**55**(6):495

[58] Brisca G, Garbarino F, Carta S, Palmieri A, Vandone M, Severino M, et al. Increased childhood peripheral facial palsy in the emergency department during covid-19 pandemic. Pediatric Emergency Care. 2020;**36**(10): e595-e596

[59] Kerstens J, Deschuytere L, Schotsmans K, Maréchal E. Bilateral peripheral facial palsy following asymptomatic covid-19 infection: A case report. Acta Neurologica Belgica. 2021; **121**(3):815-816

[60] Andreozzi V, D'arco B, Pagliano P, Toriello A, Barone P. Bilateral facial palsy after COVID-19 vaccination. Neurological Sciences. 2022: 1-11

[61] Inui R, Fujiwara S, Kohara N, Kawamoto M. Post covid-19 bilateral facial nerve palsy. Internal Medicine. 2022;**61**(2):241-243

[62] Estakhr M, Tabrizi R, Ghotbi Z, Shahabi S, Habibzadeh A, Bashi A, Borhani-Haghighi A. Is facial nerve palsy an Early Manifestation of COVID-19? A Literature Review. The American Journal of the Medical Sciences. 2022;**364**(3): 264-273. DOI: 10.1016/j.amjms.2022. 04.010. Epub 2022 Apr 14. PMID: 35429449; PMCID: PMC9007824

[63] Egilmez OK, Gündoğan ME, Yılmaz MS, Güven M. Can covid-19 cause peripheral facial nerve palsy? SN comprehensive. Clinical Medicine. 2021; **3**(8):1707-1713

[64] Martínez-Angeles WL, González-Reynoso O, García-Ramírez MA. Facial palsy estimation algorithm. In: Rosado-Mendez IM, Hernández-Bojórquez, Morales-Barcenas JH, Galavis PE, Porras-Chaverri MA, editors. AIP Conference Proceedings. Vol. 2348. Merida, Mexico: AIP Publishing LLC; 2021. p. 050035

Chapter 3

Comprehensive Rehabilitation of Patients with Facial Expression Asymmetry and Synkinesis with Botulinum Toxin Type A and Monofilament Mesothreads

Leniza Mingazova, Elena Karpova, Olga Orlova and Ada Artemenko

Abstract

Facial neuropathy is a lesion of the facial nerve of various nature happening at different anatomical levels, which is manifested by unilateral paralysis or paresis of the facial muscles and is complicated by synkinesis and contractures of the paretic muscles. The leading clinical symptom of this disorder is mimic asymmetry, which occurs as a result of a violation of the neuromuscular balance of both hemifaces (weakness on the side of the lesion and hypertonicity on the contralateral side). Understanding the special functional state of the unaffected hemiface made it possible to develop a pathogenetically substantiated method for the treatment of mimic asymmetry. The effect of botulinum toxin type A on the muscles of the healthy hemiface contributes to a better restoration of the motor activity of the affected muscles and the symmetry of the face. Implantation of monofilament mesothreads in the facial area was used to correct synkinesis. We have proposed a method that creates a rigid mesh frame using mesothreads between the skin and the muscles of facial expression in the area of synkinesis. This led to a significant decrease in the severity of clinical symptoms, a decrease in the frequency and amplitude of involuntary muscle contractions in the face.

Keywords: facial expression asymmetry, botulinum toxin type A, hypertonicity of contralateral muscles of facial expression, synkinesis, monofilament mesothreads

1. Introduction

The face has a unique nervous system. The nervous system of the face is a single synergistic system that combines both hemifaces [1–5]. Clinical observations show that pathological processes in the face are most often unilateral (Bell's palsy, trigeminal neuralgia, hemifacial spasm, etc.) [2–7]. However, in recent years, the question of the influence of the contralateral conditionally healthy hemiface in the pathological process has been actively studied [1–4, 8]. The lesion of the muscles of facial expression in facial neuropathy is also considered as a bilateral process, which involves the nervous system of both hemifaces. Besides the weakness of the muscles innervated by the facial nerve on the affected hemiface, there is an absolute hypertonicity of the muscles of facial expression of the healthy hemiface [1–4, 9]. Normally, in facial neuropathy the healthy hemiface is used for the comparison. However, a special functional state of the contralateral side, manifested by increased muscle tone, is one of the causes of facial expression asymmetry (static and dynamic) [3, 8–10]. An EMG analysis of the muscle tone of the face in the "healthy" hemiface revealed a statistically significant increase in bioelectrical activity (BEA) in patients with facial nerve neuropathy in comparison to the control group ($p < 0.05$) [1, 11]. The data obtained allow us to assert that the true over action of muscles of facial expression is formed on the "healthy" side. Activation of the contralateral side is a maladaptive response and requires therapy [1–4, 8–10]. We have used the method to influence muscle hypertonicity of the healthy hemiface in neuropathy of the facial nerve using local injections of botulinum toxin type A. Synkinesis (Greek. *syn* – together and *kinesis* – movement) is the most common complication of the facial neuropathy. Joint movements, in the form of involuntary contractions of the facial muscles that occur when performing basic facial expressions, are observed [12–14]. A patient's quality of life significantly reduces due to the synkinesis. The treatment of synkinesis is very difficult due to the lack of a positive effect of a traditional pharmacotherapy. A local injection of botulinum toxin type A in the area of synkinesis can bring a good but temporary effect [11, 14]. However, the weakness of muscles of facial expression, which develops at the same time, causes a significant frustration in patients and creates discomfort. A joint work of neurologists and plastic surgeons allowed us to propose a method for correcting synkinesis using monofilament mesothreads, which are commonly used in esthetic practice.

2. Comprehensive rehabilitation of patients with facial expression asymmetry

2.1 The use of botulinum toxin type A in patients with facial expression asymmetry

The main task of botulinum toxin therapy of facial expression asymmetry in neuropathy of the facial nerve is to influence the hypertonicity of the muscles of the healthy hemiface by muscle relaxation. The increased activity of the muscles of the contralateral (healthy) hemiface is considered to be a mechanism for pathological compensation of the functional motor deficit on the side of the lesion and may prevent or slow down the process of recovery of facial expression activity [1–4]. As a result of the treatment, after some time (10–14 days), we can observe how the affected muscles restore their functions. This contributes to the regression of facial expression asymmetry [1–4, 9]. We observed two groups of patients. In group I, there were patients in the acute phase of Bell's palsy (within 1 month after the onset of the disease), who deliberately refused corticosteroid therapy due to various reasons (diabetes mellitus, osteoporosis, poor tolerance to corticosteroids in history). Thus, monotherapy of Bell's palsy with botulinum toxin type A was carried out. Group II included patients with facial asymmetry in the late phase of Bell's palsy. The duration of the disease in this group of patients ranged from 3 months to 19 years.

The Sunnybrook Facial Grading Scale (SFGS) was used to assess facial symmetry and synkinesis, while the facial asymmetry was assessed using the House-Brackmann

Facial Nerve Granding Sale scale (1985), which consists of six levels. The first level corresponds to the normal function of the facial nerve, and the sixth level corresponds to its complete dysfunction. Static asymmetry was assessed by the displacement of the denervated muscles in relation to the central line due to the traction of the muscles of facial expression of the unaffected hemiface. Dynamic asymmetry was assessed according to several criteria: blinking frequency (video recording was made during a conversation with a doctor), muscle activity during articulation, and facial expression tests. Clinically, in all patients on the side of the lesion, there were observed narrowing of the palpebral fissure, shortening of the zygomatic and buccal muscles, drooping of the ala of the nose, mouth angle, nasal tip deviation, and displacement of the midline of the lips toward the lesion.

2.1.1 Method of administration of botulinum toxin type A in facial expression asymmetry

To correct (weaken) the pulling effect of the active muscles of the "healthy" hemiface, we perform sequential injections of the frontal, glabellar, periorbital areas, the nasal bridge, the nasolabial fold, the middle of the face, the perioral area, and chin on one side of the face. The target muscles are determined by the facial expression tests (to raise your eyebrows up, to frown, to squint, to "wrinkle" your nose, to show your teeth, to purse your lips). The most active areas of the muscles are injected. After applying local anesthesia and treating the skin with an antiseptic, the patient is given local injections of botulinum toxin type A.

The following treatment protocol was used: 100 units of botulinum toxin type A (botulinum toxin type A complex – hemagglutinin) is reconstituted with 2.0 ml of sodium chloride injection at a concentration of 9 mg/ml (0.9%). In this case, a reconstituted colorless solution is obtained with a concentration of 5 units in 0.1 ml. The solution is injected using a 1 ml syringe with a 30 G needle. In total, 1.25–2.5 units of the drug is injected into one injection point.

Subcutaneous injections are administered in the following areas of the unaffected hemiface:

1. frontalis and glabellar muscles (total 3–4 points, 1.25 units in each point), corrugator muscle (total 1–2 points, 5 units in the head of the muscle, 1.25 units in the tail of the muscle, if necessary), procerus muscle (total 1–2 points with 1.25 units) – **Figures 1** and **2**;

2. periorbital area (only 4–5 points with 1.25 units, in the area of the upper eyelid the drug is injected into the pretarsal portion of orbicularis oculi muscle) – **Figure 3**

3. the midface, the nasal bridge, the nasolabial fold – nasalis muscle (1 point with 1.25 units), levator labii superioris muscle (1 point with 1.25 units), zygomaticus minor muscle (1–2 points with 1, 25 units), zygomaticus major muscle (1–2 points with 1.25 U) – **Figure 4**

4. perioral area – orbicularis oris muscle (only 1–2 points with 1.25 units), m. depressor anguli oris (1 point with 1.25 units), depressor labii inferioris muscle (total 1–2 points with 1.25 units) – **Figure 5**

5. mentalis area – mentalis muscle (only 1–2 points with 1.25 units).

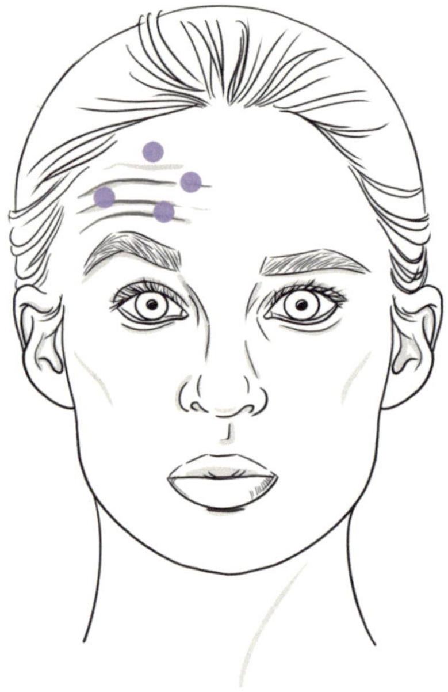

Figure 1.
Injection pattern of botulinum toxin type A in the frontal region.

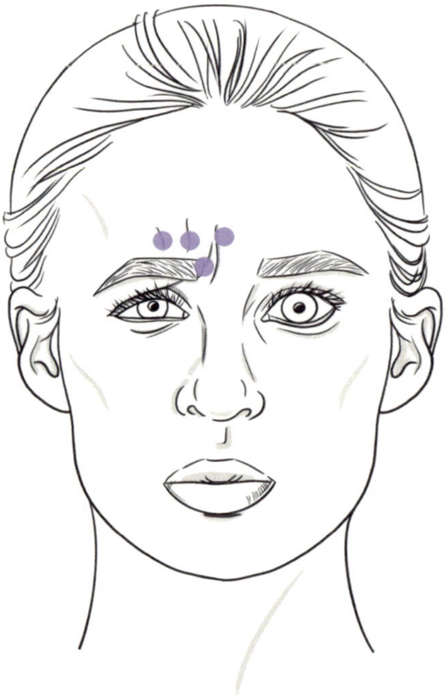

Figure 2.
Injection pattern of botulinum toxin type A in the glabellar region.

The number of injected points on the face, on average, is 15–20. During the procedure, the patient sits on a chair, resting their head against the wall. Patients sign a voluntary informed consent for medical diagnostic and treatment procedures.

DOI: http://dx.doi.org/10.5772/intechopen.106694

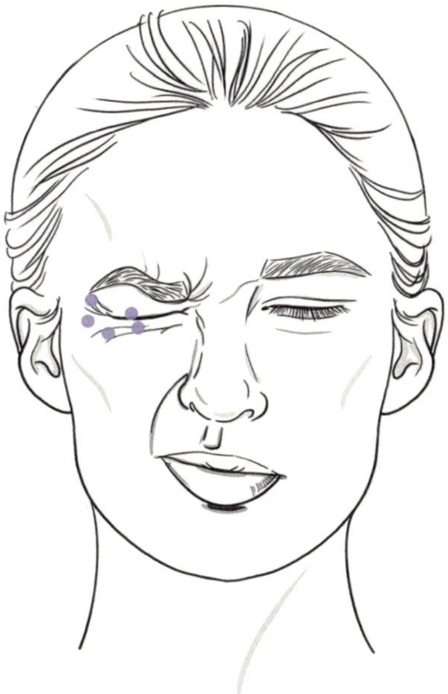

Figure 3.
Injection pattern of botulinum toxin type A in the periorbital region.

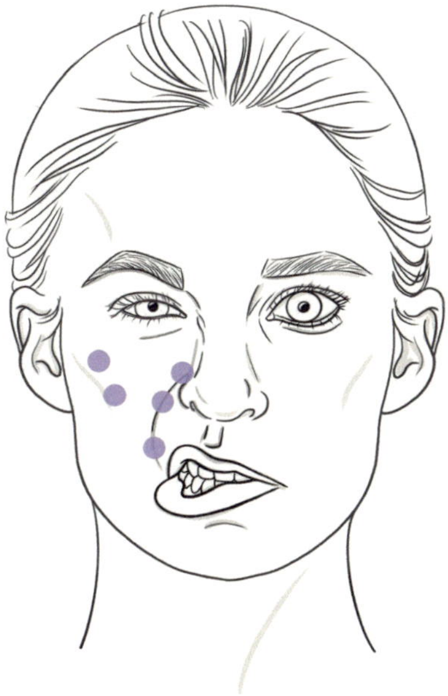

Figure 4.
Injection pattern of botulinum toxin type A in the midface.

2.1.2 Results of botulinum toxin therapy on facial expression asymmetry

Within 7–10 days after botulinum toxin type A injections, a muscle relaxant effect occurs as a reduction of muscle activity on the "healthy" hemiface and a decrease in the displacement of denervated muscles in relation to the central line of the face.

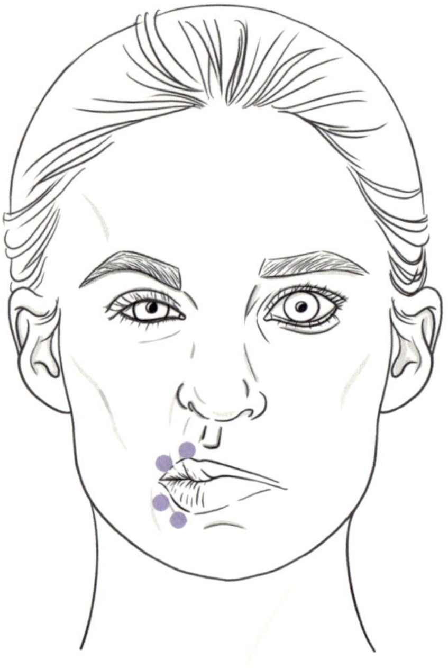

Figure 5.
Injection pattern of botulinum toxin type A in the perioral region.

Patients begin to notice a tendency of facial symmetry restoration and then a gradual activity in the denervated muscles. According to our observations, an earlier recovery is observed in the orbicularis oculi muscle, manifested in lagophthalmos regression, making it possible to close the eye, which in turn is important for the eyeball protection. Following, the activity of nasalis muscle and levator labii superioris muscle is restored. The asymmetry of the smile function is the latest to get restored, due to the slow recovery of the activity of the zygomaticus major and minor muscles and the orbicularis oris muscle.

Patients of group I showed the better recovery dynamic due to the treatment. Fourteen days after the injection of botulinum toxin type A, patients of group I showed the average decrease of score on the House-Brackmann scale by 1.85 times ($p < 0.05$), while in group II patients' score dropped only by 1.1 times ($p > 0.05$). After 1 month the improvement in patients of group I was 2.6 times ($p < 0.05$), and in group II it was 1.5 times ($p < 0.05$). The general condition of the facial muscles in patients of group I, assessed using the Sunnybrook Facial Grading System, was 3.0 times better than in patients of group II ($p < 0.01$). It is important to note that in all subscales (symmetry of rest, symmetry of voluntary movements, synkinesis), the indicators in patients of group I were better than in group II. The dynamics of symptoms of static and dynamic facial asymmetry was also more distinct in patients of group I. Patients of group II showed a less noticeable dynamics, which prompted repeated injections of botulinum toxin type A (every 3–4 months for 1–3 years). Normally, a single injection of botulinum toxin type A is sufficient for patients of group I. The ultimate effect is observed after 1 month after the injections. We observed that the muscles of the affected hemiface get restored well enough to begin to "pull" the muscles of the "healthy" hemiface, denervated by botulinum toxin, toward themselves, which is an important detail. In such a case, a temporary asymmetry occurs on the opposite side (**Figures 6–25**). The patients get informed about this phenomenon prior to the treatment. The effect of botulinum toxin gets ceased, approximately, within 3–4 months. During this period, paretic muscles significantly restore their activity. Thus, the data obtained indicate a higher efficacy of botulinum toxin therapy in patients in the acute phase of Bell's palsy.

We should note that in some patients suffering from the facial expression asymmetry, there was observed a poor recovery of the paretic muscles. This was registered both among patients of group I (20%) and among patients of group II (38%).

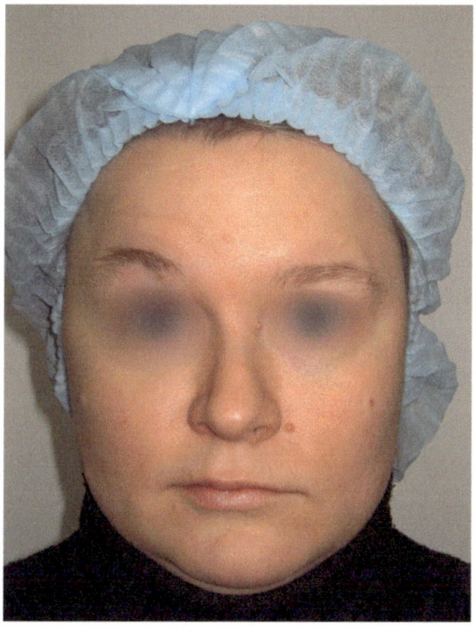

Figure 6.
Bell's palsy. Patient B. before injections.

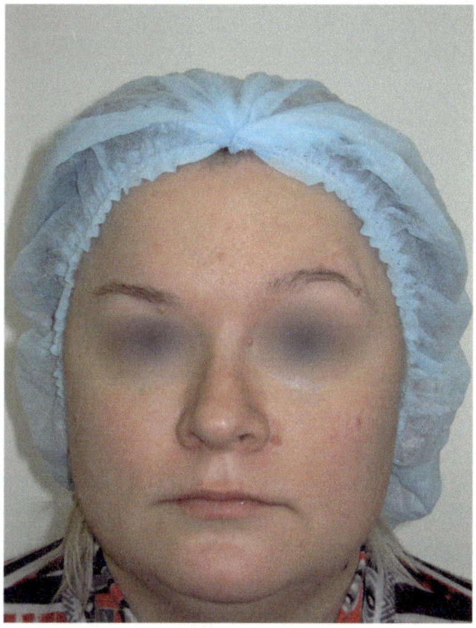

Figure 7.
Patient B, 1 month after injection.

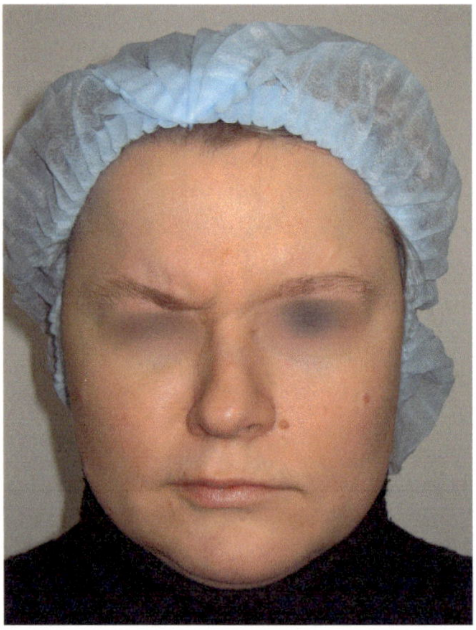

Figure 8.
Bell's palsy. Patient B. before injections.

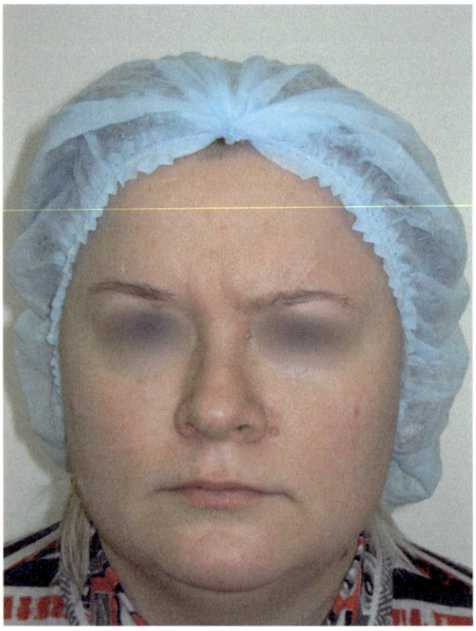

Figure 9.
Patient B, 1 month after injection.

Unfortunately, we were unable to identify predictors of the efficacy of botulinum therapy for patients with facial neuropathy. However, given the data obtained on a statistically significant improvement of the condition of the majority of patients studied, we believe that every patient with a damaged facial nerve should be offered to receive botulinum toxin injections. Other adverse events of botulinum therapy include temporary dryness of the eye on the side of the injection, which may occur after the drug is injected into the orbicularis oculi muscle.

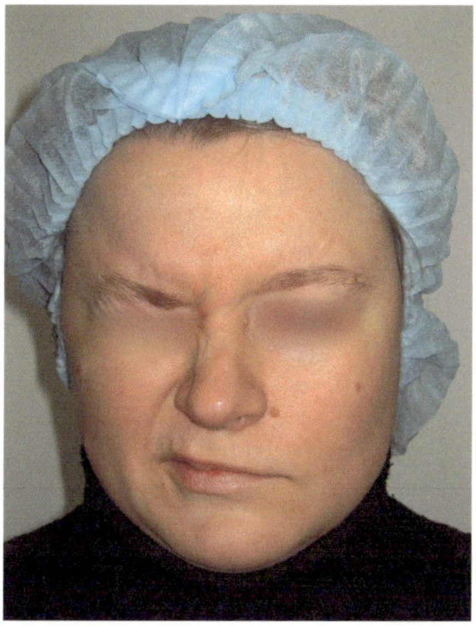

Figure 10.
Bell's palsy. Patient B. before injections.

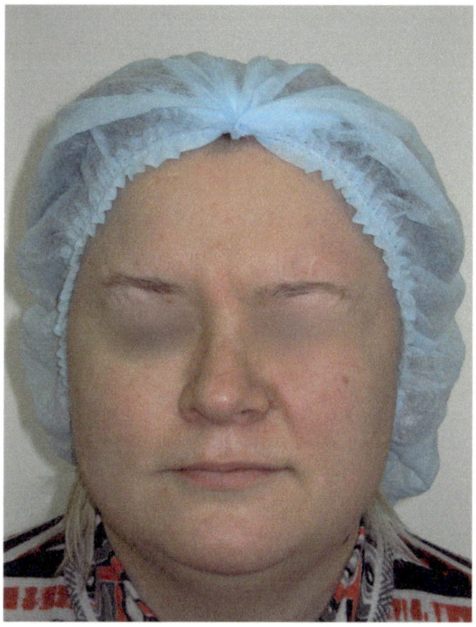

Figure 11.
Patient B, 1 month after injection.

2.2 The use of monofilament mesothreads for the treatment of synkinesis

Patients, suffering from the lesion of the facial nerve, develop the synkinesis and contractures on the affected side of the face in 4–6 months amid already existing weakness of muscles of facial expression. Synkinesis is involuntary movements of the facial muscles of one muscle group in response to voluntary movements of another muscle group of the face [12, 13, 15]. Currently, there are three hypotheses for the occurrence of synkinesis. The theory that has received the greatest recognition is that

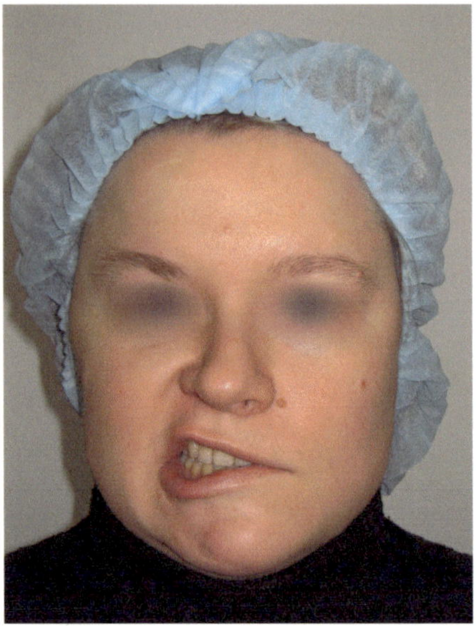

Figure 12.
Bell's palsy. Patient B. before injections.

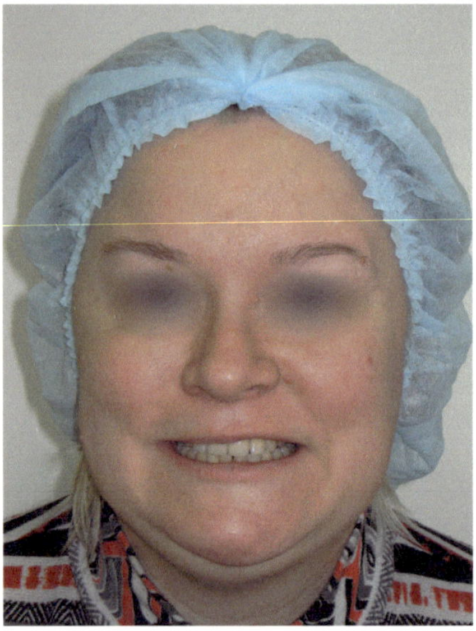

Figure 13.
Patient B, 1 month after injection.

after damage, axons undergo aberrant regeneration forming the innervation of those muscles they had not previously been innervated. The second potential pathological mechanism involves ephaptic signaling, in which neighboring axons in the affected area stimulate each other, probably as a result of loss of myelin sheath. Finally, some studies indicate the possibility of a central mechanism of synkinesis origin as a result of overexcitation of the motor nucleus of the facial nerve [14, 15].

In clinical practice, the most common cases of synkinesis are oculo-oral (movement of the zygomaticus major and minor muscles, the orbicularis oris muscle while

DOI: http://dx.doi.org/10.5772/intechopen.106694

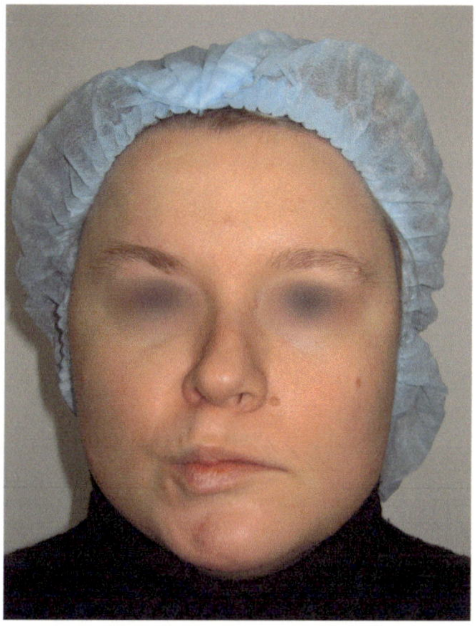

Figure 14.
Bell's palsy. Patient B. before injections.

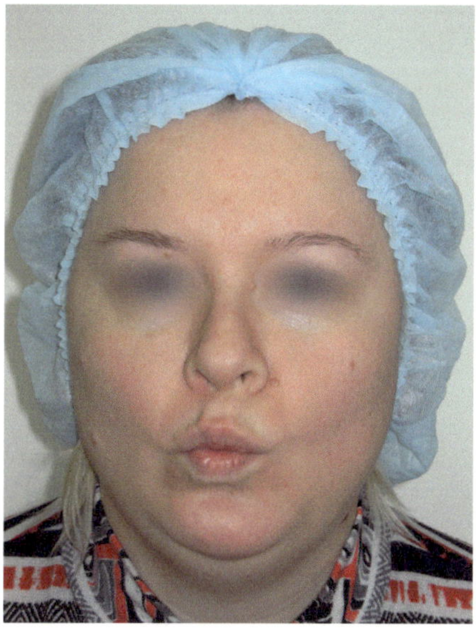

Figure 15.
Patient B, 1 month after injection.

the arbitrary closure of the palpebral fissure) and oral-ocular (narrowing of the palpebral fissure during mouth movement). To diagnose oculo-oral synkinesis, we use the "frequent blinking" test, when the patient is asked to blink frequently. In this case, there is a contraction of the zygomatic, buccal and perioral muscles observed. To diagnose oral-ocular synkinesis, the "u-e" or "b-p" test is used, which allows to trace the narrowing of the palpebral fissure on the side of the lesion, which manifests in the patient "winking" during a conversation.

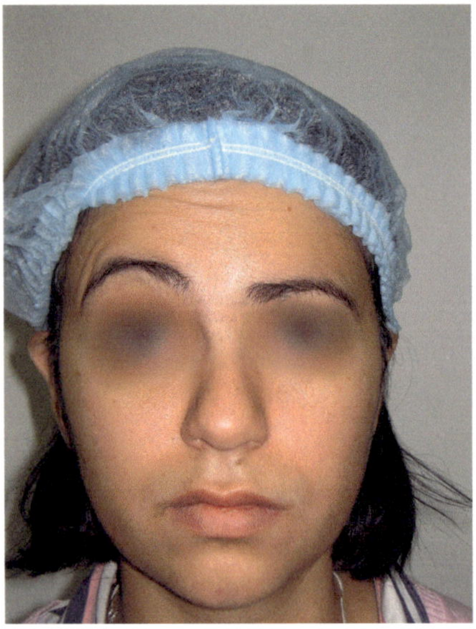

Figure 16.
Bell's palsy. Patient A. before injections.

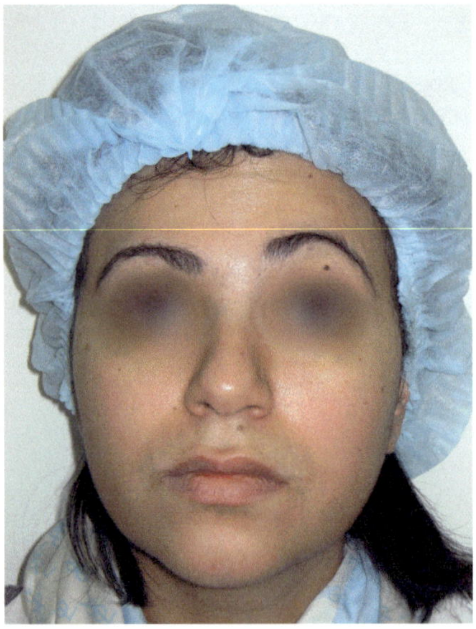

Figure 17.
Patient A., 1 month after injection.

Due to the fact that synkinesis is usually manifested by interchanging hyper- and hypokinesis zones, the applied methods of treatment should be aimed both at suppressing excessive muscle activity, depending on the area of the face, and at restoring mobility. Such physiotherapy methods as physiotherapy exercises, massage, electrical stimulations are very arduous and often do not bring the desired results, because they do not influence the pathological "chain of synkinesis," which is defined by the sequence of involvement of involuntary muscle contractions on the affected side in response to voluntary movement [12, 15]. Botulinum toxin type A is used to selectively suppress the

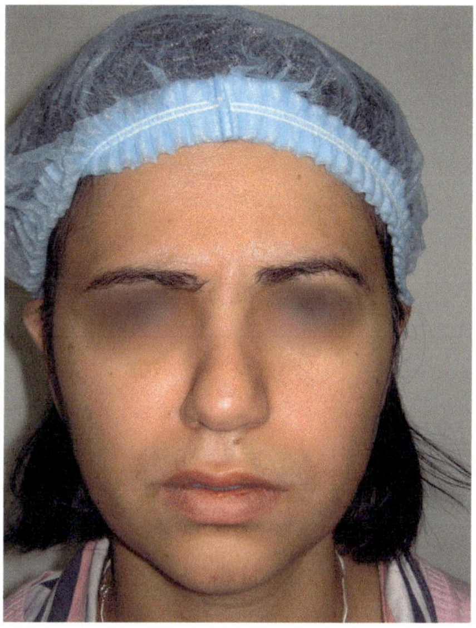

Figure 18.
Bell's palsy. Patient A. before injections.

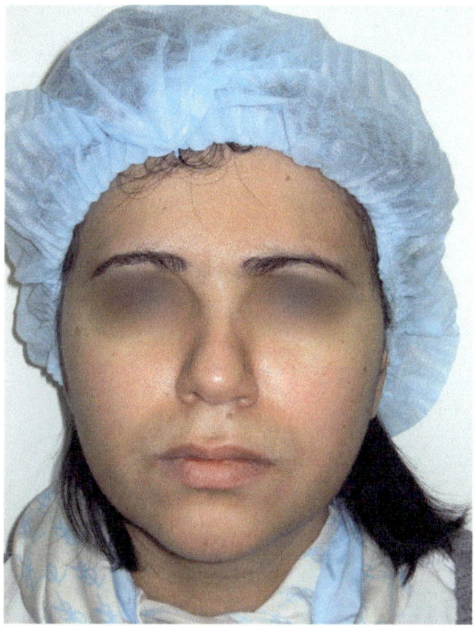

Figure 19.
Patient A., 1 month after injection.

activity of muscle fibers and is effectively used to correct synkinesis [11, 14]. However, after botulinum toxin therapy, temporary weakness of the facial muscles on the affected side may develop, which aggravates the asymmetry and causes frustration (anxiety) in patients. They start feeling as if the symptoms of the disease have reappeared, which makes many of them to refuse subsequent injections. Additionally, the effect of injections is short term (2–3 months). There are also known methods of surgical correction of synkinesis [12, 16], but they require the excision of areas of synkinesis and hospitalization in a surgical department. This can lead to persistent weakness of facial muscles and the formation of muscle contractures [11, 14].

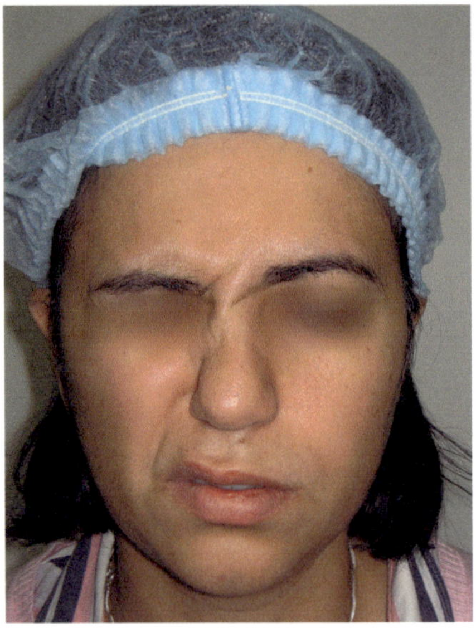

Figure 20.
Bell's palsy. Patient A. before injections.

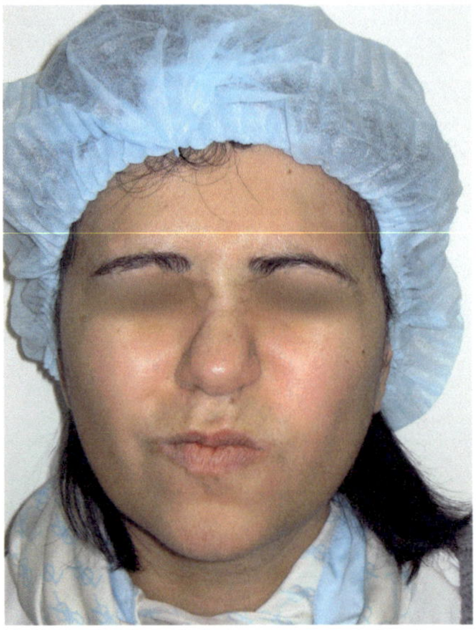

Figure 21.
Patient A., 1 month after injection.

We observed two groups of patients with Bell's palsy. All patients had oculo-oral and oral-ocular synkinesis, which developed within a year after the disease. The first group of patients received injections of botulinum toxin type A in the areas of synkinesis, while the second group of patients underwent implantation of monofilament mesothreads. The severity of pathological synkinesis was assessed using the Synkinesis Assessment Questionaire (SAQ, 2007).

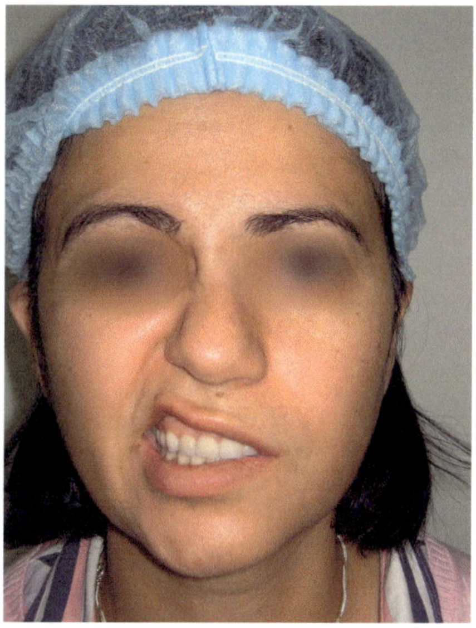

Figure 22.
Bell's palsy. Patient A. before injections.

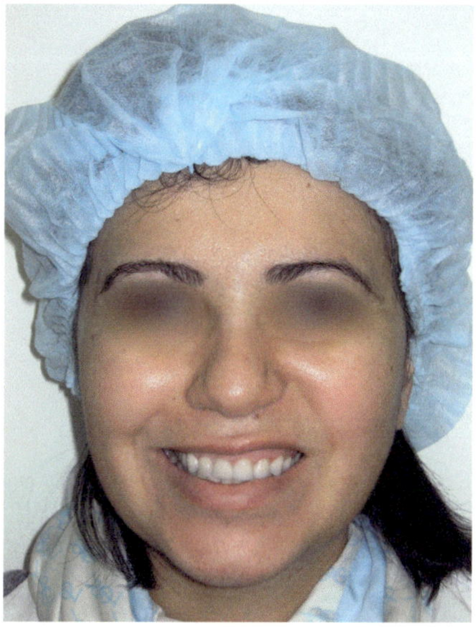

Figure 23.
Patient A., 1 month after injection.

2.2.1 Method of implantation of monofilament mesothreads to treat synkinesis

Monofilament mesothreads are among the minimally invasive rejuvenation procedures in esthetic medicine, which makes it possible to improve the involutional manifestations of aging. Mesothreads got this name due to their small diameter, comparable to the diameter of a needle for mesotherapy. These threads are used to modify

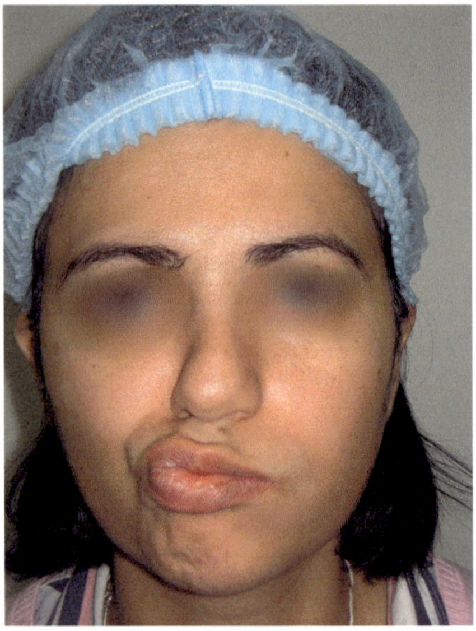

Figure 24.
Bell's palsy. Patient A. before injections.

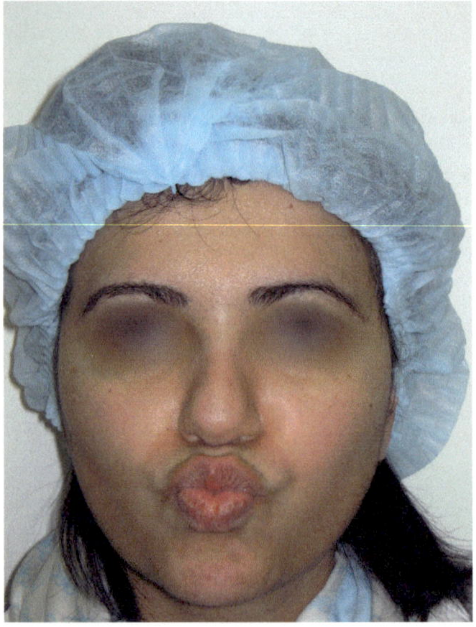

Figure 25.
Patient A., 1 month after injection.

involutional changes in the skin and ptosis of the soft tissues of the face. The visible lifting effect of the soft tissues is determined by creation of a rigid frame consisting of a large number of mesothreads and new collagen fibers forming around them [17, 18]. Clinically, this is manifested by a decrease in the severity of wrinkles and folds and an increase in skin density and elasticity [17, 18]. Mesothreads are completely bioresorbable, often made from polydioxanone - a hypoallergenic, non-toxic material that undergoes biodegradation in 180–240 days, which gives a long-term preservation effect up to 1.5–2 years. Mesothreads are applied in different age groups. In patients younger than 30 years old, it is used to prevent aging of the skin, in the older age groups, it is used to reposition the soft tissues of the face [17, 18].

There has been some data documented about the use of polydioxanone threads in combination with botulinum toxin injections for the treatment of the facial expression asymmetry [19]. The authors used the implantation of toothed threads in the subcutaneous plane along the intended trajectory in patients with unilateral sagging of the face in the late period of facial nerve neuropathy. The authors implanted patients with unilateral sagging of the face in the late period of facial nerve neuropathy with cogged threads in the subcutaneous layer along the planned trajectory. At the same time, local injections of botulinum toxin type A were performed to treat contralateral hypertrophy and ipsilateral synkinesis. As a result, the symmetry of the face got improved. Due to the lifting effect with the help of threads, there was a rejuvenation of the sagging hemiface observed, which occurs as a result of prolonged paralysis of the muscles of facial expression [19].

In our work, we used a completely different approach. We used smooth, monofilament threads (short 3–4 cm, non-cogged threads) in the affected hemiface to correct synkinesis.

The proposed method allows creating a rigid frame-mesh between the skin and muscles of facial expression, which helps to counteract their pathological contraction. The "target" for the implantation of threads is actively contracting muscle bundles. Usually, they are located in the periorbital region, along the nasolabial fold, in the projection of the modiolus and mentalis region. Synkinesis in the periorbital region manifests in muscle contractions in the infraorbital margin, the lateral part of the orbit, the superciliary arch (in the projection of corrugator muscle), as well as in the upper eyelid region. It is not possible to install threads in the upper eyelid region in the projection of levator palpebrae superioris muscle due to the high risk of thread displacement into the orbital region and muscle injury even when implanted superficially. Therefore, the use of mesothreads to treat synkinesis in the upper eyelid, inferior to the orbital rim, is impossible due to the high risk of complications. Threads are installed in the subcutaneous layer attached to the posterior layer of the dermis in the area of synkinesis, between the skin and muscles (**Figure 26**). The injection site for the introduction of the thread is at a distance of 2–3 cm in each direction from the synkinesis. The threads are implanted at a distance of 1–1.5 mm from each other and in the form of mutually intersecting lines (five threads horizontally and five threads perpendicular or at an angle). The crossing point of the threads should be in the zone of synkinesis (**Figure 27**). The thickness and length of the thread are selected depending on the area of treatment. The qualification and experience of a plastic surgeon who performs the implantation of mesothreads are key in the successful procedure. Patients were informed about ongoing medical diagnostic and treatment procedures. During the visit, each patient signed a voluntary informed consent.

2.2.2 Results of treatment of synkinesis with monofilament mesothreads

In patients of group I (who received botulinum toxin therapy), the effect appeared only 7–10 days after the administration of the drug. The amplitude and frequency of synkinesis in patients of group II (who were treated with mesothreads) decreased immediately after the completion of the procedure. A significant effect of implantation of mesothreads was also registered 7–10 days after the procedure. The amplitude and severity of synkinesis in the "u-e," "b-p" test significantly decreased. Patients noted that they managed to communicate with other people easily. The interlocutors stopped peering,

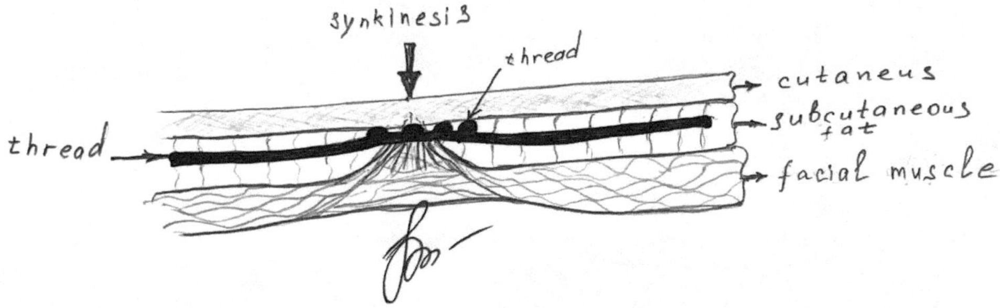

Figure 26.
Position of the threads for the treatment of synkinesis.

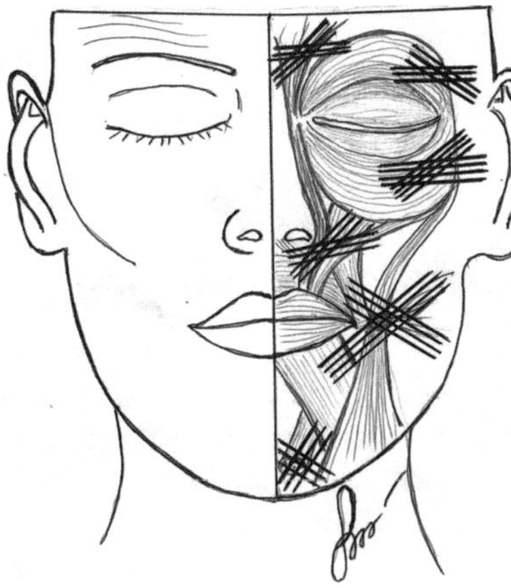

Figure 27.
Potential areas for the implantation of monofilament mesothreads in the synkinesis region.

trying to discern the involuntary movements of the muscles of the face in patients, which significantly increased patients' self-esteem, improved the quality of life.

In 1, 3, 6, and 12 months after the procedures, the general condition of the facial muscles of patients of group II, assessed using the SFGS scale, was 2.0, 2.3, 2.4, and 1.9 times better than in patients of group I ($p < 0.01$). In 50% of cases, the positive effect of mesothreads on synkinesis persisted even after 1.5–2 years.

Thus, a comparative analysis of two methods for treatment of motor synkinesis showed the best result in the group of patients who received monofilament mesothreads. We observed a significant decrease in the severity of clinical symptoms, manifested in a decrease of the frequency and amplitude of involuntary muscle contractions in the face.

The proposed method has limitation. It is likely to develop a hematoma at the injection sites of mesothreads (especially in the periorbital region). There is a risk of rejection of the threads within the first 2–3 days (due to the extremely superficial introduction). In such a case, it is important to remove the thread, holding it by the tip. It is likely to experience pain after thread implantation (within 1–2 days), as well as a relatively long rehabilitation period (up to 10 days).

In the later period (6–12 months), it is likely to have a migration of threads and the formation of a ligature fistula. There have been no such complications in our practice.

3. Remarks

1. Pathological process of facial nerve neuropathy affects both hemifaces. On the affected side, a pronounced motor deficit becomes apparent. On the contralateral side, hyperactivity of muscles of facial expression is determined.

2. Botulinum toxin treatment for facial expression asymmetry, which affects the neuromuscular apparatus of the "healthy" hemiface, helps to restore the balanced work of both hemifaces. This creates favorable conditions for the correct joint interaction of facial muscles, increasing the motor activity of the facial muscles of the affected hemiface.

3. To treat motor facial synkinesis, we created a mesh-frame of monofilament mesothreads between the skin and facial muscles, and new collagen fibers forming around them. This helped to significantly decrease the clinical symptoms, which were expressed by a decrease in the frequency and amplitude of involuntary muscle contractions in the face.

4. Conclusion

Thus, the signs of facial expression asymmetry in facial nerve neuropathy include weakness of the facial muscles innervated by the affected facial nerve, as well as hypertonicity of the facial expression muscles of the healthy hemiface. The proposed method of injections of botulinum toxin type A into hyperactive facial expression muscles of the unaffected ("healthy") hemiface in case of facial nerve neuropathy contributes to the formation of a balance between both hemifaces and the joint work of the nervous structures of the face. Botulinum toxin therapy is a pathogenetically substantiated method of restoring facial symmetry. Due to this method, it is possible to achieve an increase in the motor activity of the muscles of facial expression of the affected hemiface both in the acute phase of Bell's palsy, and with remaining effects in the long-term period. This method is also applicable for the treatment of facial expression asymmetry of another etiology, for example, as a result of an iatrogenic injury (found in cosmetology, plastic surgery, and maxillofacial surgery). The efficacy of botulinum toxin therapy is explained by other impacts besides the local muscle relaxant effect of botulinum toxin type A. It is known that the action of botulinum toxin type A causes peripheral deafferentation. This suggests a neuroplastic effect on the segmental, suprasegmental structures of the facial nerve system when performing injections in the face.

The use of the proposed method for the treatment of pathological synkinesis using monofilament mesothreads showed a good result. The creation of a mesh-frame between the facial muscles and the skin in the area of involuntary muscle contractions reduces the external manifestations of synkinesis. The use of monofilament mesothreads makes it possible to obtain a longer and more stable clinical effect, which is manifested by a decrease in the severity and amplitude of pathological muscle contractions of facial muscles, even in 2 years after the treatment.

Acknowledgements

The authors would like to thank Amina Mukhambetova for translating this article into English and Elizaveta Soikher for creating anatomical illustrations.

Conflict of interest

None of the other authors listed have any commercial associations or financial disclosures that might pose or create a conflict of interest.

Author details

Leniza Mingazova[1*], Elena Karpova[2], Olga Orlova[1] and Ada Artemenko[1]

1 Department of Nervous Diseases, Post-Graduate Education Institute, Sechenov University, Moscow, Russian Federation

2 Department of Dermatological Diseases and Cosmetology, Pirogov State Medical University, Moscow, Russian Federation

*Address all correspondence to: mleniza@mail.ru

References

[1] Saksonova E, Orlova O, Kurenkov A. Mint: The functional asymmetry of the facial neuromotor apparatus in patients with facial nerve neuropathy and its treatment with botulinum toxin type A lantox. Zhurnal Nevrologii i Psikhiatrii imeni S.S. Korsakova. 2013;**113**(10):29-35. (In Russ.)

[2] do Nascimento Remigio AF, Salles AG, de Faria JC, Ferreira MC. Mint: Comparison of the efficiency of onabotulinumtoxinA and abobotulinumtoxinA at the 1:3 conversion ratio for the treatment of asymmetry after long-term facial paralysis. Plastic and Reconstructive Surgery. 2015;**135**:239-249

[3] Kim KJ. Mint: Contralateral botulinum toxin injection to improve facial asymmetry after acute facial paralysis. Otology and Neurotology. 2013;**34**(2):319-324. DOI: 11.1097/mao.0b013e31827c9f58

[4] de Sanctis PC, de Sanctis SD, Pecora C, et al. Botulinum toxin type A to improve facial symmetry in facial palsy: A practical guideline and clinical experience. Toxins (Basel). 2021;**13**(2):159. DOI: 10.3390/toxins13020159

[5] Xiao L, Pan Y, Zhang X, Hu Y, Cai L, Nie Z, et al. Mint: Facial asymmetry in patients with hemifacial spasm before and after botulinum toxin A treatment. Neurological Sciences. 2016;**37**:1807-1813

[6] Yuksel B, Genc F, Yaman A, Goksu EO, Ak PD, Gomceli YB. Mint: Evaluation of stigmatization in hemifacial spasm and quality of life before and after botulinum toxin treatment. Acta Neurologica Belgica. 2019;**119**:55-60

[7] Xiao L, Pan L, Li B, Zhou Y, Pan Y, Zhang X, et al. Mint: Botulinum toxin therapy of hemifacial spasm: Bilateral injections can reduce facial asymmetry. Journal of Neurology. 2018;**265**:2097-2105

[8] Pourmomeny AA, Pourali E, Pourmomeny AA CA, et al. Mint: Neuromuscular retraining versus BTX-A injection in subjects with chronic facial nerve palsy, A Clinical Trial. Iran Journal of Otorhinolaryngology. 2021;**33**(116):151-155. DOI: 12.22038/ijorl.2021.41305.2347

[9] Hamidian Jahromi A, Hamidian KP, Jahromi A, et al. Mint: Contralateral facial botulinum toxin injection in cases with acute facial paralysis may improve the functional recovery: Where we stand and the future direction. World Journal of Plastic Surgery. 2021;**10**(2):89-92. DOI: 10.29252/wjps.10.2.89

[10] Shokri T, Azizzadeh B, Ducic Y, Shokri T, et al. Mint: Modern management of facial nerve disorders. Seminars in Plastic Surgery. 2020;**34**(4):277-285. DOI: 10.1055/s-0040-1721824

[11] Akulov MA, Orlova OR, Orlova AS, Usachev DJ, Shimansky VN, Tanjashin SV, et al. Mint: IncobotulinumtoxinA treatment of facial nerve palsy after neurosurgery. Journal of the Neurological Sciences. 2017;**381**:130-134

[12] Shinn JR, Nwabueze NN, Du L, Patel PN, Motamedi KK, Norton C, et al. Mint: Treatment patterns and outcomes in botulinum therapy for patients with facial synkinesis. JAMA Facial Plastic Surgery. 2019;**21**(3):244-251. DOI: 10.1001/jamafacial.2018.1962

[13] Markey JD, Loyo M. Latest advances in the management of facial synkinesis. Current Opinion in Otolaryngology & Head and Neck Surgery. 2017;**25**(4):265-272. DOI: 10.1097/moo.0000000000000376

[14] Couch SM, Chundury RV, Holds JB. Mint: Subjective and objective outcome measures in the treatment of facial nerve synkinesis with onabotulinumtoxin A (botox). Ophthalmic Plastic and Reconstructive Surgery. 2014;**30**:246-250. DOI: 10.1097/iop.0000000000000086

[15] Maria CM, Kim J. Individualized management of facial synkinesis based on facial function. Acta Oto-Laryngologica. 2017;**137**(9):1010-1015. DOI: 10.1080/00016489.2017.1316871

[16] Wamkpah NS, Jeanpierre L, Lieu JEC, Del Toro D, Simon LE, Chi JJ, et al. Mint: Physical therapy for iatrogenic facial paralysis: A systematic review. JAMA Otolaryngology and Head and Neck Surgery. 2020;**146**(11):1065-1072. DOI: 15.1001/jamaoto.2020.3049

[17] Choe WJ, Kim HD, Han BH, Kim J. Mint: Thread lifting: A minimally invasive surgical technique for long-standing facial paralysis. HNO. 2017;**65**:910-915

[18] Kim B, Seungmin O, Jung W. The Art and science of thread lifting. In: Based on Pinch Anatomy. Singapore: Springer Nature Singapore Pte Ltd.; 2019. p. 242. DOI: 10.1007/978-981-13-0614-3

[19] Bhatnagar A, Rai R, Kumar S, Mitra B, Chopra A, Singh GK, et al. Safety and efficacy of restoring facial symmetry using polydioxanone thread face lift technique in patients with facial palsy. The Journal of Clinical and Aesthetic Dermatology. 2022;**15**(2):26-29

Chapter 4

Reanimation of Mouth Corner with Free Gracilis Muscle Flap

Serdar Nasir and Alaz Cirak

Abstract

Gracilis muscle is the most commonly used muscle in facial paralysis. Although the use of the contralateral buccal branches with the sural nerve graft as the recipient nerve provides spontaneous smiling, the main disadvantage is the weak contraction due to insufficient muscle innervation. Although the masseter nerve is a chewing muscle, it can be used as a recipient nerve to provide a strong contraction. However, postoperative adaptation of the brain is required to ensure spontaneous smiling. In this article, I will evaluate the results of the postoperative third-year results of 11 patients with partial thickness gracilis muscle. I carried on the masseter recipient nerve for oral corner reanimation in facial paralysis.

Keywords: facial paralysis, cranial nerves, facial nerve injuries, facial reanimation, free gracilis muscle flap

1. Introduction

In complete facial paralysis, the effected parts of the patients' face are frontalis muscle, muscles of facial expressions, and platysma muscle in the neck. The inability that troubles patients the most is the paralysis of the muscles on the effected side that pull the mouth corner vectorally outward from the center of the face during the act of smiling. Zygomaticus major muscle and minor muscle, which pull the upper lip upward and which are the main muscles that function during smiling, combined with rhisorius muscle, which pull the side of the lip outward, create the function of smiling. In a study it has been found that children smile 400 times and adults smile 20 times in a day and the importance of the action of smiling in people's lives in introducing themselves to their social environment has been shown [1]. In unilateral facial paralysis, an asymmetrical view is formed during smiling due to the lack of function in the muscles described above and in bilateral facial paralysis (Moebius syndrome, etc.), a motionless face is formed, which causes an apathic face appearance. Attempts on gaining the function of smiling constitute the main basis in facial reanimation operations, which are operations that aim to recreate the function of the effected muscles in cases of facial paralysis. Attempts on the muscles that close the eyelids are the second most frequent operations. Functional muscle transfer is done in attempts to recreate function of smiling. In this article, I am going to mention my experiences on single session gracilis muscle transfer in which masseter nerve is used as the recipient nerve.

IntechOpen

2. Materials and method

In this study, 11 patients of at least 3 years of follow-up (between 2011 and 2019) are included. Following preauricular incision, a pouch is created by lifting the skin flap at the mouth corner upward and downward. After the outer edge of masseter muscle is found and after a back parallel line is drawn starting from 1 to 1.5 cm away from the zygomatic arch, a point is marked on that line 3–3.5 cm away from tragus. Masseter nerve is found by parallel dissection to muscle fibers between superficial and deep lobes of masseter muscle, approximately at 1.5 cm deep of superficial musculoaponeurotic system (SMAS) [2]. Nerve is dissected at its full length, the branch that goes to deep lobe is preserved, and the superficial branch is determined as the recipient nerve. On inner side of the thigh, adductor longus muscle is palpated, a parallel incision to that muscle is made, and gracilis muscle is found positioned medially to adductor longus muscle (**Figure 1**). After dissection of the pedicle, markings on the muscle, 3 cm apart from each other, are made with absorbable sutures, which are going to define the entrance site of the central predicle (**Figure 2**). Branch of the obturator nerve to gracilis muscle is tracked to the site of origin from the main nerve

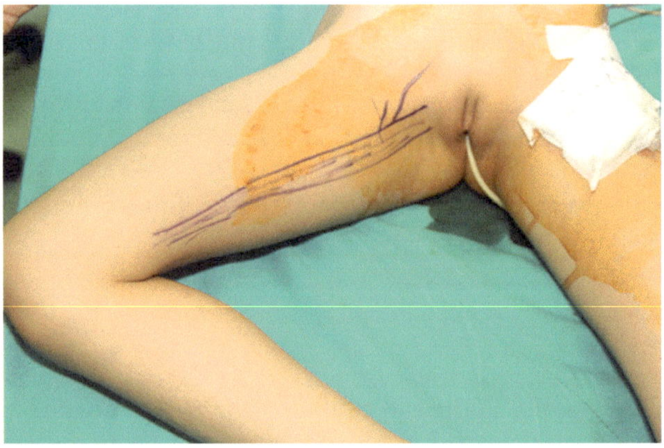

Figure 1.
View of the gracilis muscle and its pedicle drawn on skin.

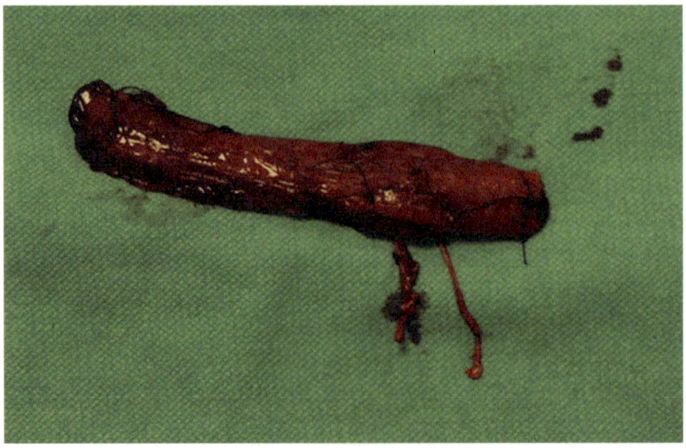

Figure 2.
Gracilis free muscle flap marked at 3 cm intervals.

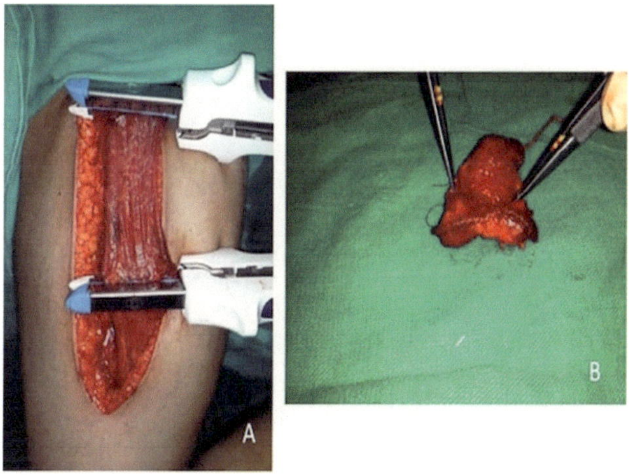

Figure 3.
Removal of the muscle flap with straight intestinal stapler.

body. About 1/3–2/3 anterior segment of the muscle, 2–3 cm longer than the distance between zygomatic arch and mouth corner, is taken using a straight intestinal stapler (**Figure 3**). The size of the segment that is going to be used is determined according to the entrance site of the pedicle on the muscle. First of all, to technically facilitate the procedure, nerve of the gracilis muscle flap is repaired and sutured to the recipient masseter nerve. Then, flap is transferred to facial artery and vein, which had been prepared as recipient vessels. Upper end of the muscle is sutured to zygomatic arch with 2/0 Polydioxanone (PDS). Distal end of the muscle is divided in three parts: upper part is sutured to the upper side of the lip and to the base of nose, lower part is sutured to the side of the lower lip, and middle part is sutured to the mouth corner. After the operation, patient's mouth corner is sutured as a static strap, in a position that muscles stay tight and constricted, symmetrical to the contralateral side. A drain is placed next to the pedicle, without completely closing the preauricular incision, bleeding control on the end of the muscle and circulatory control with Doppler Ultrasound are performed. Patients are immobilized for 5 days in bed. No anticoagulants were used and only be used local heating with floor lamp. After day 5, with observation of normal circulation following mobilization, preauricular incision is closed. Average time that patients start to feel the first muscle contractions is observed to be around 2 months. After contractions begin, Transcutaneous Electrical Nerve Stimulation (TENS) device is used on patients for 20 minutes four times in a day. The traction of the mouth corner is started to be observed around 6–8 months on average. Patients' muscle power being increased, maximum muscle strength is achieved approximately 1.5–2 years on average. After patients start to pull the lip corner, physiotherapy is started. Advices of practicing control on smiling movements with a mirror, guidance on patients' social lives, which may lead to all day smiling, and advice of watching a comedy movie every other day were made to patients.

3. Results

Pictures of patients were taken after patients were informed about their pictures were to be used and published in scientific papers. Verbal and written consent has been

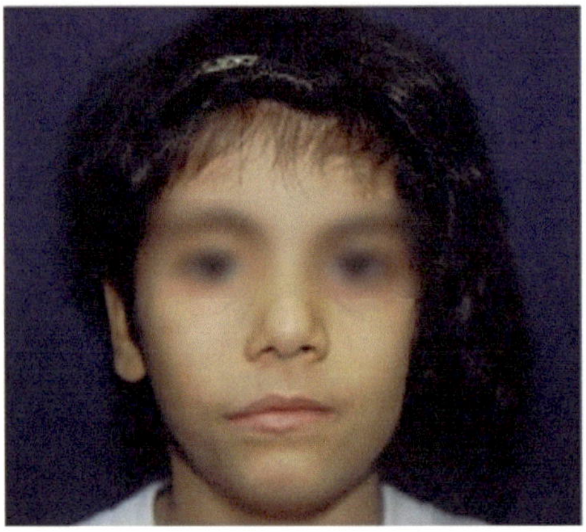

Figure 4.
Preoperative view of the patient.

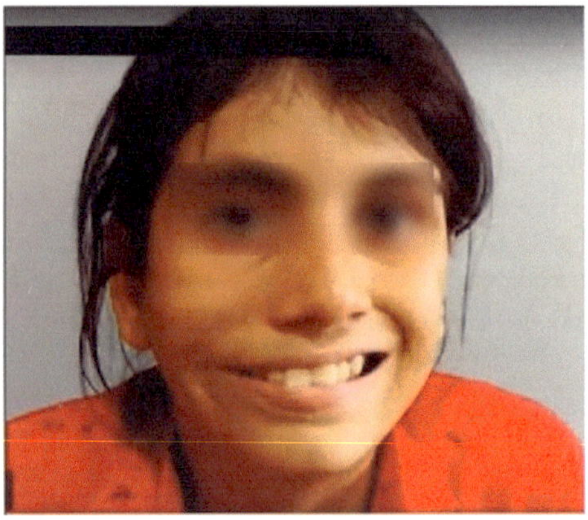

Figure 5.
View of the patient 8 years after the operation.

acquired from patients regarding the use of their pictures in publications. No flap loss is observed. On eight of the patients, symmetrical smiling to the contralateral side is observed (**Figures 4** and 5), on two of the patients, a pull 1–1.5 cm less than the contralateral side is observed. However, because of patient satisfaction, no muscle plication attempts aiming augmentation of traction of the lip corner were made. A swollen appearance on the face is observed on six of the patients due to muscles; however, since patients are still on follow-up period, a flap thinning procedure has not been performed.

4. Discussion

Although the most common choice is use of gracilis muscle in reanimation of smiling muscles in facial paralysis [3], free muscle transfers such as serratus anterior muscle, latissimus dorsi muscle, extensor digitorum brevis muscle, and pedicled muscle transfers such as temporalis muscle transfers have been used.

In free muscle transfers, the contralateral facial nerve with use of nerve grafts, ipsilateral hypoglossal nerve (12th Cranial Nerve (CN)), ipsilateral accessory nerve

(11th CN), or the ipsilateral masseter nerve, which is one of the motor branches of fifth CN, can be used as the recipient nerves. In the cases where the contralateral facial nerve is used as the recipient nerve, when an impulse is generated toward the contralateral side, it passes on the nerve graft and causes contraction of the transferred muscle, which in the end causes a "spontaneous smile" on the effected side. This situation is not possible in cases where other cranial nerves except facial nerve on the same side are used as the recipient nerve. In the beginning of cases, which are used CV as recipient nerve, in order to generate smiling function on the operated side, the patient needs to think of an action, which will cause their chewing muscles to work. In the studies carried out, it has been shown that masticatory center and smiling center in the brain are located close to each other and with certain exercises accessory neural pathways will be generated between these two centers [4]. Therefore, it has been stated that smiling function will be performed with use of these pathways when patients want to smile. Some studies state that simultaneous stimulation of masticatory center causes action on transferred muscle to generate smiling action, during the stimulation of the smiling center. It has been stated that success of the operation is increased with younger patient. When transfer to the masseter nerve operations is performed on patients who were in childhood, spontaneous smiling is achieved at advanced ages approximately 80% of the patients, compared with 50–80% of the patients when the operation is done in older ages [5, 6]. There are important exercises that the patient and the physiotherapist need to perform in order the neural pathways to be created. Patients are advised to smile constantly in their social lives. This includes daily life advices from greeting everyone in the most appropriate way to social lives, to trying to use every opportunity throughout the day to smile. Patients are advised to watch a comedy movie on alternate days. Furthermore, one of the most important practices is exercises to be done in front of a mirror. The goal of these exercises is to increase patients' comprehension of the traction strength on the transferred side during smiling and to equalize their smile with the contralateral side. Therefore, patients are going to make their brains learn the traction power of the transferred muscle, and they are going to equalize the strength on both sides of their face during smiling. To start these exercises, it is necessary to wait until the maximum traction strength of the transferred muscle is achieved and revision operations regarding muscle traction and tension are completed. On my cases, I start external electrical stimulus by using TENS devices when patients feel the first contraction on the transferred muscle, although a clinically visible contraction has not been achieved. I suggest these external stimuli are given in 20 minute sessions every 3 hours. Therefore, I believe that the number of new neuromuscular junctions is increased and direct muscle stimulation is provided during muscle innervation period, which prevents muscle atrophy. There is a direct proportion between the number of neurons in the recipient nerve and contraction strength of transferred muscle. With increased number of neurons in the recipient nerve, the number of neurons, which reach the transferred muscle and cause contraction, is increased. In valuable studies carried out, it is stated that buccal branch of the facial nerve contains approximately 834+/−285 neurons. When these neurons are used at the paralyzed side with a sural nerve graft, the axons budded from the recipient nerve need to pass through two nerve coaptation sites through the nerve graft. In studies carried out, number of the neurons of buccal nerve is observed to be around 100–200 after these neurons pass through the nerve graft and reach the transferred muscle. This situation is because number of neurons of the recipient nerve is few and because neurons pass through two coaptation sites. The branch of the masseter nerve that is used as the recipient nerve contains 1542+/−291 neurons [2, 7], which is much greater than buccal branch of the facial nerve. Other benefit of using the masseter nerve is, since neurons are going to pass through a single nerve coaptation site, the decrease in the number of neurons that reach the transferred muscle is going to be less compared with when buccal branch is used as the recipient nerve. In a study, it is shown that the number of neurons pass to the obturatory nerve from masseter nerve is 10–15 times greater than the neurons pass through sural nerve graft. In my clinical practice, in the beginning I used buccal branches as the recipient nerves. However, because I observed muscle traction strength was fairly weak and because a second session was needed, I have started to transfer partial thickness gracilis muscle to the masseter nerve as the recipient nerve with a single session operation. The second frequent complaint of patients who had free muscle transfer is the unaesthetic view of the patients' faces during contraction caused by excessive swelling, following the most common complaints, which are about traction strength [8]. This is the reason during removal of the flap from donor site, I use 1/3–2/3 of the muscle according to entrance site of the pedicle8. I use straight intestinal staplers to remove the muscle flap to be transferred from the main muscle. Therefore, ends of the muscle flap stay together preventing separation of fibers at the ends of the flap. These titanium staplers facilitate fixation of proximal end of the flap to zygomatic arch and by preventing fibers from scattering staplers facilitate division of the distal end to three parts, one for upper lip, one for lower lip, and one for mouth corner. Therefore, fixation of muscle fibers to sides of lips and mouth corner, which is among the most important parts of the operation, can easily be done with the help of staplers. I suggest that if a flap thinning operation is being planned, it should be performed at late stages after the operation. Because I believe in the long terms if the muscle is fixated to the recipient site properly and soundly, it adapts well and a thinning operation is not going to be necessary. I believe that most of the permanent swellings during muscle contraction are caused by poor fixation of the muscle to lip corner or to the zygomatic arch or detachment of the muscle from fixation sites because of poor wound healing or weak adhesion of the muscle. However, if none of the problems stated above exists and swelling during contraction is observable, a thinning operation to the nearest parts of the muscle to the skin can be performed very carefully. It has to be kept in mind that as a result of a careless procedure, contractions of the transferred muscle can be totally lost.

5. Conclusions

As a result, I believe reanimation of smiling function in facial paralysis with one session partial thickness free gracilis muscle flap with the masseter nerve as the recipient nerve is superior to other techniques despite some disadvantages regarding spontaneous smiling.

Conflict of interest

The authors declare no conflict of interest.

Author details

Serdar Nasir and Alaz Cirak*
Reconstructive and Aesthetic Surgery Department, Hacettepe University Faculty of Medicine Plastic, Ankara, Turkey

*Address all correspondence to: cirakalaz@gmail.com

References

[1] Weker M. Smile and lie? Why we are able to distinguish false smiles from genuine ones. In: Evers D, Fuller M, Runehov A, Sæther KW, editors. Issues in Science and Theology: Do Emotions Shape the World? Cham: Springer; 2016. pp. 59-71. DOI: 10.1007/978-3-319-26769-2_5

[2] Borschel GH, Kawamura DH, Kasukurthi R, Hunter DA, Zuker RM, Woo AS. The motornerve to the masseter muscle: An anatomic and histomorphometric study to facilitate its use in facial reanimation. Journal of Plastic, Reconstructive & Aesthetic Surgery. 2012;**65**(3):363-366

[3] Roy M, Corkum JP, Shah PS, Borschel GH, Ho ES, Zuker RM, et al. Effectiveness and safety of the use of gracilis muscle for dynamic smile restoration in facial paralysis: A systematic review and meta-analysis. Journal of Plastic, Reconstructive & Aesthetic Surgery. 2019;**72**(8):1254-1264

[4] Hontanilla B, Cabello A. Spontaneity of smile after facial paralysis rehabilitation when using a non-facial donor nerve. Journal of Cranio-Maxillo-Facial Surgery. 2016;**44**(9):1305-1309

[5] van Veen MM, Dusseldorp JR, Quatela O, Baiungo J, Robinson M, Jowett N, et al. Patient experience in nerve-to-masseter-driven smile reanimation. Journal of Plastic, Reconstructive & Aesthetic Surgery. 2019;**72**(8):1265-1271

[6] Bianchi B, Ferri A, Ferrari S, Copelli C, Salvagni L, Sesenna E. The masseteric nerve: A versatile power source in facial animation techniques. The British Journal of Oral & Maxillofacial Surgery. 2014;**52**(3):264-269

[7] Coombs CJ, Ek EW, Wu T, Cleland H, Leung MK. Masseteric-facial nerve coaptaiton-an alternative technique for facial nerve reinnervation. Journal of Plastic, Reconstructive & Aesthetic Surgery. 2009;**62**(12):1580-1588

[8] Greene JJ, Tavares J, Guarin DL, Jowett N, Hadlock T. Surgical refinement following free Gracilis transfer for smile reanimation. Annals of Plastic Surgery. 2018;**81**(3):329-334

Chapter 5

Management of Bell's Palsy with Phototherapy

Lok Yan Joanne Cheng, Tai Hong Andrew Lung and Shu Yan Ng

Abstract

Bell's palsy (BP) is a common condition; its incidence rate has increased during the COVID-19 pandemic. The standard treatment for facial nerve palsy includes corticosteroids alone or in combination with antiviral agents. However, the treatment is contraindicated in some patients, including hypertensive or diabetic patients. Also, the medication combination may result in inadequate recovery when complementary and alternative approaches are indicated. This chapter reviewed the literature on managing BP with different types of photobiomodulation (PBM) therapies. Fourteen papers were included. The results show that despite the different kinds of photo energy used, varying laser parameters, and the heterogeneity of patients, the outcome of PBM was similar among studies. Of interest is that acute and subacute BP respond more favorably to PBM than chronic cases. Hence, it is suggested to apply PMB as a complementary treatment in the early stage of the disease to enhance the recovery rate of BP patients. However, the risk of bias in these studies was relatively high. Therefore, further randomized, double-blind placebo-controlled studies are needed to determine the effectiveness of PBM in treating BP.

Keywords: bell's palsy, facial paralysis, low-level laser therapy, infrared laser, phototherapy, COVID-19

1. Introduction

Bell's palsy (BP) is a common condition presented to physicians. It affects 23 people in every 100,000 yearly, and one in every 60–70 people will develop BP in their lifetime [1]. It is the most common acute facial lesion that unilaterally affects the facial nerve. It occurs when the facial nerve is swollen or compressed within the facial canal. The compromised facial nerve results in an array of symptoms, including temporary weakness or paralysis in the facial muscles, difficulty in mastication, loss of taste, drooping eyelid or corner of the mouth, drooling, poor closure of the eye, and pain in the auricular area. With an acute onset, the symptoms can develop within 72 hours and gradually resolve within weeks or months [2, 3]. However, around 30% of patients may not fully recover and experience residue dysfunction [2, 4].

 IntechOpen

1.1 Etiology of Bell's Palsy

With the exact cause of BP remaining unclear, a recent review summarized five potential clinical etiologies of this condition [5]:

- Anatomical difference – A smaller diameter of the internal acoustic meatus and facial canal and a thicker facial nerve are observed in BP patients [6, 7]. These anatomical differences may be a predisposing factor to facial nerve entrapment.

- Viral infection - Herpes-simplex virus type-1 (HSV-1) is commonly found in BP patients. The reactivation of the HSV-1 in latently infected patients can induce demyelination and degeneration in the facial nerve [8–10]. Besides the infection of HSV-1, an increased incidence rate has been noticed during the coronavirus infectious disease 2019 (COVID-19) pandemic. Several recent studies have discussed the potential causal relationship between vaccination or COVID-19 infection with BP [11–13].

- Autoimmune reaction – Autoimmune reaction is regarded as a possible etiology of BP, as a significantly high level of neutrophil-to-lymphocyte ratio (NLR) and pro-inflammatory cytokines level are detected in BP patients. Also, the autoimmune reaction can induce facial nerve demyelination [14, 15].

- Ischemia - Vasospasm in the stylomastoid artery may be another underlying risk in causing BP. Vasospasm induces ischemia, which can lead to periarteritis and obliterative endarteritis, which in turn can induce facial nerve sheath fibrosis, strangulating the nerve [16].

- Cold stimulation responsivity - The incidence rate of BP is higher in cold seasons [17, 18]. The subcutaneous fat may react to climate change, inducing the immune-inflammatory response and leading to acute facial nerve demyelination [19, 20].

However, the actual cause of BP remains unknown and requires further studies [5].

1.2 Relationship between COVID-19 and Bell's Palsy

Besides the unknown etiology of BP, a statistically significant higher incidence of BP is observed in 2020 compared to 2019. The increased incidence is associated with the COVID-19 pandemic [21]. A systematic review showed significant evidence that BP is the only major neurological manifestation in COVID-19 patients [12]. Another systematic review conducted by the same authors reviewed 46 COVID-19 cases. Around 70% of the cases showed complete recovery from BP symptoms, while over 20% of them had residual symptoms after combination treatment, mainly of corticosteroids and antiviral drugs [11]. Although the evidence of BP being the major neurological symptom in COVID-19 is significant, further studies are required to identify how the severe acute respiratory syndrome coronavirus 2 (SARS-CoV-2) exactly causes the neurological symptoms [11, 12].

Along with a higher risk of developing BP with COVID-19 infection, BP has also been recognized as a common adverse event after COVID-19 vaccination. A systematic review recognized BP as one of the most common adverse events after mRNA and viral vector-based immunization [13]. In addition, a study in Hong Kong reported a significantly increased risk of Bell's palsy following the vaccination of inactivated SARS-CoV-2 vaccine but not the mRNA vaccine [22]. However, another systematic review, which studied 61 vaccinated patients immunized with different vaccines, reported that more than half of the cases developed BP after vaccination. Interestingly, BP only occurs in patients who received mRNA and viral vector-based vaccines but not in inactivated SARS-CoV-2 vaccines [23].

Both COVID-19 and COVID-19 vaccination are suspected to be a potential cause of BP. However, the relationship between COVID-19 and COVID-19 vaccine on BP has yet to be determined and requires further investigation.

1.3 Prognosis

The current standard treatment for BP includes corticosteroids alone or combined with antiviral agents, although the condition is considered idiopathic. However, different studies reported conflicting results [3]. Some studies reported inadequate recovery from the treatments [24]. Around 70% of BP patients will recover spontaneously without treatment; 10–29% of patients will have persistent dysfunction in the facial nerve [24] with an 8% recurrence rate for those who had previous episodes of BP [3].

Comparing the standard treatment of corticosteroids alone or in combination with antiviral agents, the effects of corticosteroids alone are found to be no different from placebo [25], while a higher rate of full recovery is observed with the use of antiviral drugs in combination with corticosteroids [24]. The recovery rate of using corticosteroids alone was reported to be 67% while that of the combination treatment was 78% [24]. A randomized controlled trial (RCT) indicated that when the medical treatment was delayed for more than 4 days after the onset of symptoms, the treatment has no benefit to the patients [26].

However, the treatment of corticosteroids and antiviral agents is contraindicated in some patients (e.g., hypertensive or diabetic patients) [27]. Alternative and complementary therapies may thus provide other options.

Along with the standard treatment, physicians have been using other therapeutic methods, for instance, electrical stimulation, facial exercise, massage [28], acupuncture [29], and photobiomodulation (PBM) as supplementary treatments. While the effects of electrical stimulation, facial exercise and massage were insignificant [28], acupuncture treatment potentially showed some benefits in patients with BP [30]. However, exercises, electrical stimulation and acupuncture are not recommended to be used in patients with acute BP in several clinical guidelines due to the lack of good quality evidence [29].

1.4 Role of Photobiomodulation in Bell's Palsy

Among these complementary therapies, PBM is a non-invasive treatment, which has been investigated in recent years for its effect in treating BP. Of the different types of PBM, low-level laser therapy (LLLT) has been the most studied; it is effective in regenerating peripheral nerves in the preclinical study [31]. Our study investigates whether sufficient evidence supports PBM treatment in BP patients.

2. Materials and methods

Papers were searched in PUBMED, using the Boolean search operators ("Laser" AND "Bell's Palsy," "Laser" AND "Facial Palsy," "LLLT" AND "Bell's Palsy," "Infrared" AND "Bell's Palsy"), covering the year 2012 to June 2022. All titles were then screened for relevancy. Non-English articles are excluded. We include only studies conducted on humans. All types of clinical studies evaluating the effectiveness of phototherapy are included, including case reports, case series, prospective studies, and controlled clinical trials. A manual search was also undertaken from the references of the selected papers.

3. Results

We have identified fourteen relevant papers covering the use of phototherapy in the management of Bell's Palsy, including four RCTs [28, 32–34], one prospective study [35], one case series [36], and eight case reports [29, 37–43], which we review.

Our review shows that the most studied PBM is LLLT [28, 32, 33, 35, 37, 39, 40, 42, 43]. Others include high-intensity laser therapy (HILT) [29, 32, 36, 41], monochromatic infrared energy (MIRE) [38] and laser acupuncture [34]. Rubis [41] combined PBM with cervical manipulation. Alayat et al. [32] compared the effectiveness of HILT and LLLT combined with facial massage and exercise. Ordahan and Karahan [33] studied the effect of LLLT on top facial exercises. Kuzmičić et al. [29] combined HILT with acupuncture and mirror book therapy, and Shoman et al. [28] compared LLLT with electrical stimulation.

Most subjects were adults, except for a case report on a pediatric patient [37] and two case reports on adolescents [40, 42]. We categorized the papers into acute, subacute, chronic, and unspecified, according to the time patients received PBM treatments. We defined "acute" as onset within 1 week of consultation, "subacute" as one to 12 weeks, and "chronic" as cases that present for more than 3 months. We found different laser protocols were used in the studies. The number of treatments varies, from as few as two to 45. Most studies last 6 weeks, and PMB treatment was performed three times a week. Laser parameters, including wavelengths, power, power density, frequency, and energy density, also differed vastly among studies. Most studies utilized House-Brackmann Scale (HB Scale) as an outcome measure. It is a facial nerve grading system that grades upon functional impairment, ranging from I (normal) to VI (total paralysis) [44]. Facial Disability Index (FDI), a patient-rated outcome measure, was also commonly used to assess the functional disability and quality of life in patients with facial palsy [45]. The more recent studies utilized the Sunnybrook Facial Grading System (SB System), a physician-graded scale, which includes the synkinesis section. The scale permits recognition of minor improvements in the range of movement, thus helping quantify the progress feedback to patients [46]. Other outcome measures included electromyography and nerve conduction study. Please refer to the table in **Appendix 1** for detailed characteristics of the included papers.

Despite the different types of photo energy used, marked varying laser parameters, and the heterogeneity of the patients, the outcome of laser treatment was similar among the studies.

4. Discussion

A review of the search results showed that acute and subacute Bell's palsy respond favorably to PBM [32, 33, 37–42]. Chronic Bell's palsy, however, responds less satisfactory [34, 36, 38]. Therefore, PBM seems to be a good complementary treatment to the standard treatment with medication. A RCT by Shoman et al. [28] compared the effectiveness of LLLT with electrical stimulation in conjunction with medicine, facial massage, and exercise. Results showed that combination treatment with LLLT was more efficient than electrical stimulation in facial nerve regeneration, as determined by the nerve conduction velocity measurement and SB System scoring [28]. Several studies also recruited patients non-responsive to steroids and antivirals to investigate their response to PBM treatment [29, 36, 38]. Aghamohamdi et al. [35] studied 30 poorly controlled diabetic patients who did not receive other medications for the palsy, especially corticosteroids, due to their underlying disease. The results showed complete recovery in 18 patients (60%) and partial recovery in 6 patients (20%) [35], showing that LLLT could be a safe alternative approach for BP patients with other medical condition that is contraindicated to traditional medication treatment. However, more studies are warranted to justify its effectiveness.

4.1 Mechanism of actions

PBM involves the application of red and near-infrared light, with wavelengths ranging from 600 to 1000 nm, over the area of injury or lesion. It is a non-invasive and painless therapy for patients contraindicated to corticosteroids or antiviral medication treatments [32]. PMB has anti-inflammatory effects. Light absorbed by cellular photo-receptors modulates reactive oxygen species (ROS) and promotes adenosine triphosphate (ATP) formation. Moreover, it increases micro and macro-circulation, thus increasing tissues' oxygen saturation. These improve cellular metabolism and promote faster regeneration or proliferation of the damaged tissue [47]. Furthermore, PBM can photo-dissociate the nitric oxide, which inhibits mitochondrial respiration, thus reversing mitochondrial inhibition [48]. Through these mechanisms, PBM thus dilates blood vessels, improves oxygenation, and increases immune cell traffic to the targeted structure [49].

Also, laser therapy is shown to have direct beneficial effects on the regeneration of peripheral nerves in sensory and motor deficits, such as trigeminal neuralgia, herpes zoster, and sciatica. The therapy improves the recovery of injured nerves, slows motor neuron degeneration, and promotes axonal growth and myelination. The treatment can also lower the pro-inflammatory cytokine level and raise the anti-inflammatory cytokine level [32, 35, 40]. In addition, evidence shows that the HSV-1 can be effectively suppressed by PBM [50]. Laser therapy is also found to affect tissues differently depending on the prescribed wavelengths, pulse duration, energy density, delivery system, and duration of the whole treatment [32].

4.2 Parameters of PBM treatment

Of interest is that Bell's palsy responds to light therapy with vastly different parameters, which include wavelengths, power, power density, frequency, and energy density (**Appendix 2**). The wavelengths used in the different studies vary from 660 nm [37, 43] to 1064 nm [29, 32], with most of the studies using lasers with a wavelength of 830 nm [32, 33, 42]. Also, the power of the laser used differs significantly, with some using low-level laser with a power lower than 500 mW [33, 35, 42, 43] while others use high power laser (up to 3 kW) [32]. The energy density of laser applied in different studies also varies widely, from 10 J/cm^2 [32, 33, 37] to 120 J/cm^2 [39].

Existing evidence suggests that LLLT acts on the mitochondria and cell membrane chromophores to initiate the biological response [51]. Studies have suggested the possibility of using defined wavelengths for particular biological responses, hence achieving specific therapeutic effects [52, 53]. Barbosa et al. [52] compared the effects of LLLT at 660 nm and 830 nm on sciatic nerve regeneration following crushing injuries in rat models. They found that laser at 660 nm provided early functional nerve recovery compared to other groups. Another animal study by Lee et al. [53] also showed that rats with facial nerve injuries responded positively to 633 nm light, with better facial palsy scores, larger axon diameter, and higher expression of Schwann cells, but not to 804 nm light. One of our included studies used a laser at 780 nm during the early stage of treatment, aiming for a deeper penetration [37]. Starting from the fifth session, they changed to a wavelength of 660 nm to accelerate neural recovery. Alternating the two wavelengths was suggested to balance the stimulatory and inhibitory effects and avoid plateau situations due to extended use of a single wavelength [37]. However, the standardization of laser wavelength has yet to be defined, as our review showed that BP patients respond positively to different wavelengths.

One study showed that HILT is significantly more effective than LLLT in improving the symptoms of Bell's palsy [32]. In addition, HB Scale and FDI improved more with the HILT than with LLLT [32]. Kuzmičić et al. [29] reported a case of Bell's palsy, which was treated medically with corticosteroid and antivirals 18 months prior with minimal improvement. They employed HILT, acupuncture, and mirror book therapy to treat the patient for 7 weeks. Mirror book therapy is an adapted version of the mirror box method used to treat phantom pain and paralysis. It consists of a bi-fold mirror to reflect twice the unaffected patient's face so that the patient sees a full, unaffected face. The patient then performs a series of facial exercises. The intervention resulted in significant improvement of the facial palsy. The HB Scale reduced from IV to II, the SB System improved from 24/100 to 71/100, and the FDI improved from 43/200 to 173/200 [29]. The latter study did not compare the effects of HILT with LLLT. Also, the combination therapy makes it difficult to draw conclusions relating to the effectiveness of HILT in chronic Bell's palsy. Thus, whether HILT is superior to LLLT in managing Bell's palsy requires further investigation.

4.3 Irradiation area

Apart from the different parameters of the laser applied, the treatment method differed in various studies. Six studies used the laser on seven to nine points (**Figure 1**) along the facial nerve branches of the affected side [28, 32, 33, 35, 36, 41]. A laser is applied near the mastoid process in the stylomastoid foramen, where the facial nerve exits. Also, light is used on points along the facial nerve branches, including the temporal branch across to forehead, the zygomatic branch along the zygomatic arc, the buccal nerve in the middle portion of the cheek, and the mandibular branch along the chin [35, 41]. Ton et al. [34] applied lasers on the acupuncture points; seven were on the affected face, covering all the facial nerve branches, while two were on both sides of the extremities. Other than facial nerve branches, some studies irradiate

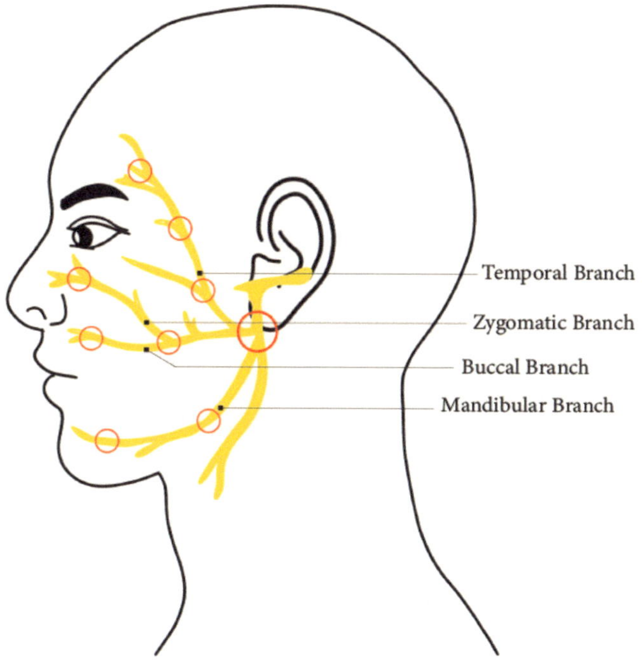

Figure 1.
Common laser application points along the facial nerves.

the facial muscles. Tanganeli et al. [39] applied laser on ten points, including the frontal, temporal, zygomatic, buccinator, lip elevator, orbicularis of the lips, lip depressor, and masseter muscles. Poloni et al. [42] only applied laser at the origin and insertion of the masseter muscle, and Fornaini et al. [40] also irradiated only the parotid gland area about the former. Bernal Rodriguez et al. [43] and Fontana and Bagnato [37] applied laser on 59 points and up to 80 points, respectively, covering all the area on the affected face. The treatment was applied to many application points because the laser beam spot is small [37, 43]. In Ng and Chu's [38] report, the four pads for MIRE therapy were placed in the post-auricular area, pre-auricular area, the temple, and the mandibular area of the affected side.

While laser therapy at the site of compression in the facial canal is understandable, the same applied over the peripheral nerve branches and muscles over the face requires further justification. Moriyama et al. [54] observed a change in gene expression in BP with the degree of facial nerve palsy. Most genes in energy and muscle categories of severe BP (HB Scale V) were downregulated, while they were upregulated in moderate BP (HB Scale III). The facial nerve conduction is largely abolished in severe BP, hence there is very little regeneration and energy production in the affected muscles and nerves [54]. This may partly explain the total or partial unresponsiveness of patients to medication [36]. On the basis of these molecular biological findings, treatment to promote muscle regeneration and energy production is hence considered. Given the ability of PBM to improve cellular metabolism and promote ATP formation [47], irradiation of the affected facial muscles and nerve branches could potentially improve the muscle regeneration and enhance the paralytic condition. Further investigations are required to compare the effects of PBM on different irradiation areas.

4.4 Timing of treatment

Also of interest is that the outcome of chronic cases is less favorable than acute and subacute cases. Ng and Chu [38] described a chronic BP case that only partially responded to MIRE. The 46 years old lady with systemic lupus erythematosus and BP for two and a half years was treated by MIRE. After 45 treatment sessions, the patient reported 50% improvement compared with baseline. Residual facial palsy was still evident [38]. Pasquale et al. [36] reported similar findings; the researchers applied HILT to a cohort of 14 patients who were non-responsive to standard treatments. The number of treatments varied from 6 to 20. Of the fourteen patients, eleven who had subacute BP improved uneventfully. However, three patients with chronic BP did not improve [36]. Similarly, Ton et al. [34] showed that LLLT did not improve chronic Bell's palsy. Seventeen chronic BP patients were randomized to treatment by laser acupuncture and sham laser. The patients were treated three times a week for 6 weeks. The outcome was measured by HB Scale, FDI, and SB System. Results showed that only HB Scale improved slightly after 3 weeks of laser acupuncture treatment compared to sham laser treatment. No significant differences were detected for HB Scale and FDI at 6 weeks between the intervention group and the sham laser treatment group [34]. One study, however, showed that LLLT improved the symptoms of chronic BP [43]. The female patient had 8 years of history of BP. LLLT treated fifty-nine points on the face of the affected side; each point was treated for 20 seconds, with 4 J per point. The patient was treated three times a week for 8 weeks. After the treatment, the HB Scale was reduced from IV to II, suggesting a partial response to LLLT [43]. Kuzmičić et al. [29] reported a chronic BP responding to combination therapy of HILT, acupuncture, and mirror book therapy.

As the outcome of these studies on chronic BP differs significantly, with some reporting favorable outcomes and others minimal changes, the use of laser therapy in chronic BP remains undetermined.

Clinically, we suggest combining phototherapy with the standard treatment to manage acute and subacute cases. Medical practitioners can refer patients to other healthcare practitioners for PBM treatment while prescribing the medications. Though chronic BP does not respond as reliably as acute and subacute cases, they should be treated for three to 6 weeks by LLLT, as some patients may respond favorably to the treatment [43]. As we are unaware of any studies on the effects of PBM on BP caused by COVID-19, we cannot provide any recommendations. However, we consider the method worth trying, particularly when the medication treatment is contraindicated.

4.5 Possibility of self-administered PBM

PBM treatments are time-consuming [55]. Clinical practice usually requires patients to return for short treatment sessions about three times a week to achieve a satisfactory result. Although laser treatments administered by trained professionals were shown to be good options for accelerating the recovery of BP [56], several studies have proposed the use of "at home" PBM devices [40]. One study prescribed a patient with a self-administered class II laser device, emitting at 808 nm and 250 mW output power, to be used twice daily, each for 15 minutes [40]. The patient simply placed the device in contact with the skin on the designated areas. After 2 weeks of treatment, the patient reported a complete recovery (HB Scale improved from IV to I) [40]. Another study reported the effects of MIRE, an array of 60 gallium aluminum arsenide light-emitting diodes, on patients with BP; it showed positive results, especially in acute patients [38]. The pads of this MIRE device could irradiate a larger area at one time compared with an infrared laser, hence reducing the need for accurate localization of facial nerve [38]. In both studies, no adverse events were reported for the devices used, and protective glasses are unnecessary, making them more favorable for self-application [38, 40]. Nevertheless, patient evaluation by practitioners before its use remains mandatory.

4.6 Contraindications and adverse effects of PBM

Phototherapy is a generally safe and non-invasive treatment. Yet, the North American Association for Laser Therapy Conference 2010 issued cautionary statements and stipulated several contraindications [48]. The operator must not point the laser beam at the eyes, and all participants in the treatment should wear appropriate safety spectacles. Practitioners must pay extra attention while operating the device as a low frequency pulsed visible light of less than 30 Hz may trigger a seizure in photosensitive and epileptic patients.

Also, it is recommended not to apply light therapy on any known primary carcinoma or secondary metastasis site, as its effects on cancer have not been elucidated [48]. Animal studies have shown PBM can be detrimental to cancer. However, other studies have shown that PBM benefits cancer treatment. It can directly damage the tumor, enhance the effects of cancer therapies, stimulate the host immune system, and increase cancer patients' survival rate [57]. In addition, if the patient is receiving chemotherapy or is defined as terminally- ill, PBM can be used to relieve the side effects of treatment and for palliative relief [48].

The evidence on the use of LLLT on cancer is limited. However, practitioners should be aware of this in the management of BP. If the patient is suffering from BP and has a known medical history of cancer somewhere else in the body, other than directly on the face, we would still consider treating the patient with LLLT. The adverse effects of the PBM are reported to be no different from placebo treatment [48].

5. Limitation of the study

Although there is an increasing number of studies investigating the effects of PBM in treating BP, the number of research in this area is still limited, and the risk of bias in these studies is relatively high. Therefore, further randomized, double-blind placebo-controlled studies are required to determine the effectiveness of PBM in treating BP, including those that are COVID-19 related.

6. Conclusion

The results of the included studies suggest that phototherapy may be a safe and promising treatment to be used in conjunction with standard medication. Earlier implementation of phototherapy could enhance the recovery rate of Bell's palsy patients. However, further high-quality studies are needed to determine its effectiveness and establish a standardized treatment protocol for this treatment option.

Conflict of interest

The authors declare no conflict of interest.

Abbreviation

BP	Bell's palsy
PBM	Photobiomodulation
LLLT	Low-level laser therapy
HILT	High-intensity laser therapy
MIRE	Monochromatic infrared energy
HB Scale	House-Brackmann Scale
FDI	Facial Disability Index
SB System	SunnyBrook Facial Grading System
HSV-1	Herpes-simplex virus type-1
NLR	Neutrophil-to-lymphocyte ratio
SARS-CoV-2	Severe acute respiratory syndrome coronavirus 2
ROS	Reactive oxygen species
ATP	Adenosine triphosphate
NO	Nitric oxide
RCT	Randomized controlled trials

A. Appendices

Stage	Paper	Study design	Sample (Patient no.; age)	Treatment	Number of sessions	Outcome measures	Outcome
Acute	Fontana and Bagnato [37]	Case report	1; 3	LLLT	11 in 3wks (4/wk. in first 2 wks)	HB Scale	Improved from Grade 5 to 1
	Ng and Chu [38]	Case report	1; 32	MIRE	19 in 6wks (daily in first 2 wks, except weekend; 3rd-5th wk., 2/wk.; after that 1/wk)	Clinical presentation	95% improvement, with mild weakness in the closure of left eyelid; Complete recovery 8 months after last treatment
	Tanganeli et al. [39]	Case report	1; 71	LLLT	10 in 6.5wks	HB Scale	Improved from Grade 5 to 1
	Fornaini et al. [40]	Case report	1; 15	"At-home PBM" class II laser	Twice a day for 2wks	HB Scale	Improved from Grade 4 to 1
Subacute	Rubis [41]	Case report	1; 40	HILT + cervical manipulation	2 in 4 days	HB Scale	Improved from Grade 5 to 1
	Alayat et al. [32]	RCT	48; 43 ± 9.8	1. HILT + facial massage and exercise 2. LLLT + facial massage and exercise 3. Facial massage and exercise	18 in 6wks (3/wk)	FDI and HB Scale	Both HILT and LLLT are more effective than the control group, with HILT showing greater improvement
	Ordahan and Karahan [33]	RCT	46; 41 ± 9.7	1. LLLT + facial exercise 2. Facial exercise	18 in 6wks (3/wk)	FDI	Combined treatment with LLLT and facial exercise therapy significantly improved FDI compared with exercise alone
	Poloni et al. [42]	Case report	1; 13	LLLT	3 in 3wks	Clinical presentation	Total recovery without recurrence after 3 years
Chronic	Ng and Chu [38]	Case report	1; 46	MIRE (Previous treatment with corticosteroid and electro-acupuncture)	45 in 9.5mths	Clinical presentation	50% improvement; condition was stable 5 months after last treatment with mild synkinesis
	Bernal Rodriguez et al. [43]	Case report	1; 25	LLLT	24 in 8wks (3/wk) Phase 1: 18; Phase 2: 6	HB Scale and electroneur-omyography	Improved from Grade 4 to 2; The amplitude of motor conduction velocity improved

Stage	Paper	Study design	Sample (Patient no.; age)	Treatment	Number of sessions	Outcome measures	Outcome
	Pasquale et al. [36]	Case series	14; 56.07 ± 15.21	HILT (Non-responsive to standard treatment of corticosteroid and acyclovir)	From 6 up to 20; Every 2 days until complete resolution	HB Scale	11 patients, with BP max. of 6 months, completely recovered. The remaining 3 patients with BP for years show no improvement.
	Ton et al. [34]	RCT	17; 1. 37.83 2. 47.75	1. Laser acupuncture 2. Sham laser	18 in 6wks (3/wk)	FDI, HB Scale, SB System, stiffness scale	A significant difference in HB score, borderline significance in SB and stiffness score, and no significant difference in FDI
	Kuzmičić et al. [29]	Case report	1; 30	HILT + acupuncture, mirror book therapy (Non-responsive to corticosteroid, facial exercises, and electrostimulation)	19 (3/wk. for 3wks, then 2/wk. for 5wks)	HB Scale, SB System, FDI	Improvement in all outcome measures HB Scale: 4/6 to 2/6 SB System: 24/100 to 71/100 FDI: 43/200 to 173/200
Un-specified	Aghamohamdi et al. [35]	Prospective study	30; ~40	LLLT	12 in 4wks (3/wk)	HB Scale, electromyography, and nerve conduction study	Complete recovery in 18 patients and partial recovery in 6 patients after 3 months.
	Shoman et al. [28]	RCT	45; ~33	1. LLLT + medication, massage, facial exercise 2. ES + medication, massage, facial exercise 3. medication, massage, facial exercise	12 in 6wks (2/wk)	Nerve conduction study, SB System	LLLT is more efficient than ES in facial nerve regeneration for Bell's palsy patients.

LLLT, low-level laser therapy; HILT, high-intensity laser therapy; MIRE, monochromatic infrared energy; PBM, photobiomodulation; ES, electrical stimulation; HB Scale, House-Brackmann Scale; FDI, Facial Disability Index; SB System, SunnyBrook Grading System; BP, Bell's Palsy.

Appendix 1.
The interventions and outcome measures of included studies.

Stage	Paper	Type of photo-energy	Wavelength (nm)	Output power (mW)	Energy density (J/cm²)	Treatment
Acute	Fontana and Bagnato[37]	LLLT	660 and 780	40–70	10–17.5	Up to 80 points; 15–30 min; 10 s/point
	Ng and Chu [38]	MIRE	890	60 mW/cm²	108	40mins
	Tanganeli et al. [39]	LLLT	808	100	120 (3.3 J/point)	10 points, 10 s/point
	Fornaini et al. [40]	"At-home PBM" class II laser	808	250	48	Twice a day, each of 15mins
Subacute	Rubis [41]	HILT	910	Up to 100,000	47.6 x 10 J	17mins; 30–60s/point
	Alayat et al. [32]	HILT	1064	Up to 3 kW	10	8 points; 7 s/point
		LLLT	830	100	10	8 points; 125 s/point
	Ordahan and Karahan [33]	LLLT	830	100	10	8 points; 2mins/point
	Poloni et al. [42]	LLLT	830	100	100	2 points; 28 s/point
Chronic	Ng and Chu [38]	MIRE	890	60 mW/cm²	108	45mins
	Bernal Rodriguez et al. [43]	LLLT	660 and 808	200	Phase 1: 40.65 Phase 2: 60.97	59 points; Phase 1: 20s Phase 30s
	Pasquale et al. [36]	HILT	808	1000	60	7 points; 60 s/point
	Ton et al. [34]	LLLT (Laser acupuncture)	810	Up to 150	45	9 points; 40/80s for local/distal acupuncture points
	Kuzmičić et al. [29]	HILT	1064	7000	80	—
Unspecified	Aghamohamdi et al. [35]	LLLT	980	334	5 J/point	9 points; 1 min/point
	Shoman et al. [28]	LLLT	850	1 W/cm²	_	8 points; 1 min/point

Appendix 2.
Laser parameters of the included studies.

Author details

Lok Yan Joanne Cheng*, Tai Hong Andrew Lung and Shu Yan Ng
Hong Kong Chiropractic College Foundation, Wan Chai, Hong Kong

*Address all correspondence to: joannecheng61@gmail.com

References

[1] Marson AG, Salinas R. Clinical evidence: Bell's palsy. Western Journal of Medicine. 2000;**173**(4): 266-268. DOI: 10.1136/ewjm. 173.4.266

[2] Baugh RF, Basura GJ, Ishii LE, Schwartz SR, Drumheller CM, Burkholder R, et al. Clinical practice guideline: Bell's palsy. Otolaryngology–Head and Neck Surgery. 2013;**149** (3_suppl):S1-S27. DOI: 10.1177/0194599813505967

[3] Tiemstra JD, Khatkhate N. Bell's palsy: Diagnosis and management. American Family Physician. 2007;**76**(7): 997-1002

[4] Prud'hon S, Kubis N. Bell's palsy. La Revue de Médecine Interne. 2019; **40**(1):28-37. DOI: 10.1016/j. revmed.2018.03.011

[5] Zhang W, Xu L, Luo T, Wu F, Zhao B, Li X. The etiology of Bell's palsy: A review. Journal of Neurology. 2020; **267**(7):1896-1905. DOI: 10.1007/s00415-019-09282-4

[6] Yilmaz HB, Safak Yalcin K, Çakan D, Paksoy M, Erdogan BA, Sanli A. Is there a relationship between Bell's palsy and internal auditory canal? Indian Journal of Otolaryngology and Head & Neck Surgery. 2015;**67**(3): 319-323. DOI: 10.1007/s12070-014-0809-0

[7] Ozan Sanhal E, Arslan H. Evaluation of the facial nerve and internal auditory canal cross-sectional areas on three-dimensional fast imaging employing steady-state acquisition magnetic resonance imaging in Bell's palsy. The Turkish Journal of Medical Sciences. 2018;**48**(3):525-530. DOI: 10.3906/sag-1707-142

[8] McCormick DP. Herpes-simplex virus as a cause of Bell's palsy. Lancet. 1972;**1**(7757):937-939. DOI: 10.1016/s0140-6736(72)91499-7

[9] Wu Y, Yang Q, Wang M, Chen S, Jia R, Yang Q, et al. Multifaceted roles of ICP22/ORF63 proteins in the life cycle of human herpesviruses. Frontiers in Microbiology. 2021;**12**:668461. DOI: 10.3389/fmicb.2021.668461

[10] Murakami S, Mizobuchi M, Nakashiro Y, Doi T, Hato N, Yanagihara N. Bell palsy and herpes simplex virus: identification of viral DNA in endoneurial fluid and muscle. Annals of Internal Medicine. 1996;**124** (1 Pt 1):27-30. DOI: 10.7326/0003-4819-124-1_part_1-199601010-00005

[11] Gupta S, Jawanda MK. Surge of Bell's Palsy in the era of COVID-19: Systematic review. European Journal of Neurology. 2022;**00**:1-18. DOI: 10.1111/ene.15371

[12] Gupta S, Jawanda MK, Taneja N, Taneja T. A systematic review of Bell's Palsy as the only major neurological manifestation in COVID-19 patients. Journal of Clinical Neuroscience. 2021; **90**:284-292. DOI: 10.1016/j. jocn.2021.06.016

[13] Sadeghalvad M, Mansourabadi AH, Noori M, Nejadghaderi SA, Masoomikarimi M, Alimohammadi M, et al. Recent developments in SARS-CoV-2 vaccines: A systematic review of the current studies. Reviews in Medical Virology. 2022:e2359. DOI: 10.1002/rmv.2359

[14] Kum RO, Yurtsever Kum N, Ozcan M, Yilmaz YF, Gungor V, Unal A, et al. Elevated neutrophil-to-lymphocyte ratio in Bell's palsy and its correlation

with facial nerve enhancement on MRI. Otolaryngology and Head and Neck Surgery. 2015;**152**(1):130-135. DOI: 10.1177/0194599814555841

[15] Yilmaz M, Tarakcioğlu M, Bayazit N, Bayazit YA, Namiduru M, Kanlikama M. Serum cytokine levels in Bell's palsy. Journal of the Neurological Sciences. 2002;**197**(1–2):69-72. DOI: 10.1016/s0022-510x(02)00049-7

[16] Grewal DS. Bell's palsy-tertiary ischemia: an etiological factor in residual facial palsy. Indian Journal of Otolaryngology and Head & Neck Surgery. 2018;**70**(3):374

[17] Spengos K, Sameli S, Stouraitis G, Kolias A, Koulouri O, Kokkinos Z, et al. Seasonal variation of Bell's palsy in Athens, Greece - A hospital-based retrospective evaluation over fifteen years. European Neurology. [cited June 13, 2022]. 2006;**55**(2):84-88. DOI: 10.1007/s12070-018-1381-9

[18] Hsieh RL, Wang LY, Lee WC. Correlation between the incidence and severity of Bell's palsy and seasonal variations in Taiwan. The International Journal of Neuroscience. 2013;**123**(7): 459-464. DOI: 10.3109/00207454.2013.763804

[19] Vielma SA, Klein RL, Levingston CA, Young MRI. Adipocytes as immune regulatory cells. International Immunopharmacology. 2013;**16**(2): 224-231. DOI: 10.1016/j.intimp.2013.04.002

[20] Huh JY, Park YJ, Ham M, Kim JB. Crosstalk between adipocytes and immune cells in adipose tissue inflammation and metabolic dysregulation in obesity. Molecules and Cells. 2014;**37**(5):365-371. DOI: 10.14348/molcells.2014.0074

[21] Zammit M, Markey A, Webb C. A rise in facial nerve palsies during the coronavirus disease 2019 pandemic. The Journal of Laryngology & Otology. 2020; **134**(10):905-908. DOI: 10.1017/S0022215120002121

[22] Wan EYF, Chui CSL, Lai FTT, Chan EWY, Li X, Yan VKC, et al. Bell's palsy following vaccination with mRNA (BNT162b2) and inactivated (CoronaVac) SARS-CoV-2 vaccines: A case series and nested case-control study. The Lancet Infectious Diseases. 2022; **22**(1):64-72. DOI: 10.1016/S1473-3099(21)00451-5

[23] Shafiq A, Salameh MA, Laswi I, Mohammed I, Mhaimeed O, Mhaimeed N, et al. Neurological immune-related adverse events after COVID-19 vaccination: A systematic review. Journal of Clinical Pharmacology. 2022;**62**(3):291-303. DOI: 10.1002/jcph.2017

[24] Kim Y, Doo JG, Chon J, Lee JH, Jung J, Lee JM, et al. Steroids plus antiviral agents are more effective than steroids alone in the treatment of severe Bell's palsy patients over 40 years of age. International Journal of Immunopathology and Pharmacology. 2021;**35**:20587384211042124. DOI: 10.1177/20587384211042124

[25] Salinas RA, Alvarez G, Ferreira J. Corticosteroids for Bell's palsy (idiopathic facial paralysis). Cochrane Database of Systematic Reviews. 2004; (4):CD001941. DOI: 10.1002/14651858.CD001942.pub2

[26] Hato N, Matsumoto S, Kisaki H, Takahashi H, Wakisaka H, Honda N, et al. Efficacy of early treatment of Bell's palsy with oral acyclovir and prednisolone. Otology & Neurotology. 2003;**24**(6):948-951. DOI: 10.1097/00129492-200311000-00022

[27] Tamez-Pérez HE, Quintanilla-Flores DL, Rodríguez-Gutiérrez R, González-González JG, Tamez-Peña AL. Steroid hyperglycemia: Prevalence, early detection and therapeutic recommendations: A narrative review. World Journal of Diabetes. 2015;**6**(8): 1073-1081. DOI: 10.4239/wjd.v6.i8.1073

[28] Shoman A, Hassan A, Kassab A. A study on the effect of 850 nm low-level diode laser versus electrical stimulation in facial nerve regeneration for patients with Bell's Palsy. ORL: Journal for Otorhinolaryngology and Its Related Specialties. 2022:1-8. DOI: 10.1159/000521789 [Online]

[29] Kuzmičić S, Pavić A, Vidović A, Kuzmičić N, Bećir B, Parlov M, et al. Chronic Bell's Palsy literature review and case report: Are there any rehabilitation strategies available? Hrvatski časopis zdravstvenih znanosti. 2022;**2**(1):59-63. DOI: 10.48188/hczz.2.1.4

[30] Zhang R, Wu T, Wang R, Wang D, Liu Q. Compare the efficacy of acupuncture with drugs in the treatment of Bell's palsy: A systematic review and meta-analysis of RCTs. Medicine. 2019; **98**(19):e15566. DOI: 10.1097/MD.0000000000015566

[31] Kneebone WJ. Enhancement of nerve regeneration by therapeutic laser. Practical Pain Management. 2010;**10**(4): 70-72

[32] Alayat MSM, Elsodany AM, El Fiky AAR. Efficacy of high and low level laser therapy in the treatment of Bell's palsy: A randomized double blind placebo-controlled trial. Lasers in Medical Science. 2014;**29**(1):335-342. DOI: 10.1007/s10103-013-1352-z

[33] Ordahan B, Karahan AY. Role of low-level laser therapy added to facial expression exercises in patients with idiopathic facial (Bell's) palsy. Lasers in Medical Science. 2017;**32**(4):931-936. DOI: 10.1007/s10103-017-2195-9

[34] Ton G, Lee LW, Ho WC, Tu CH, Chen YH, Lee YC. Effects of laser acupuncture therapy for patients with inadequate recovery from bell's palsy: Preliminary results from randomized, double-blind, sham-controlled study. Journal of Lasers in Medical Sciences. 2021;**12**(1):e70. DOI: 10.34172/jlms.2021.70

[35] Aghamohamdi D, Fakhari S, Farhoudi M, Farzin H. The efficacy of low-level laser therapy in the treatment of bell's palsy in diabetic patients. Journal of Lasers in Medical Sciences. 2020; **11**(3):310-315. DOI: 10.34172/jlms.2020.52

[36] Pasquale C, Utyuzh A, Mikhailova MV, Colombo E, Amaroli A. Recovery from idiopathic facial paralysis (Bell's Palsy) using photobiomodulation in patients non-responsive to standard treatment: A case series study. Photonics. 2021;**8**(8):341-352. DOI: 10.3390/photonics8080341

[37] Fontana CR, Bagnato VS. Low-level laser therapy in pediatric bell's palsy: Case report in a three-year-old child. The Journal of Alternative and Complementary Medicine. 2013;**19**(4): 376-382. DOI: 10.1089/acm.2011.0531

[38] Ng SY, Chu MHE. Treatment of Bell's Palsy using monochromatic infrared energy: A report of 2 cases. Journal of Chiropractic Medicine. 2014; **13**(2):96-103. DOI: 10.1016/j.jcm.2014.06.010

[39] Tanganeli JPC, de Oliveira SSI, da Silva T, Fernandes KPS, Motta LJ, Bussadori SK. Complete and fast recovery from idiopathic facial paralysis using laser-photobiomodulation. Case

Reports in Dentistry. 2020;**2020**: 9867693. DOI: 10.1155/2020/9867693

[40] Fornaini C, Meng Z, Merigo E, Rocca JP. "At-Home" photobiomodulation: A new approach for Bell's Palsy treatment. Case Reports in Neurological Medicine. 2021;**2021**: 5043458. DOI: 10.1155/2021/5043458

[41] Rubis LM. Chiropractic management of Bell palsy with low level laser and manipulation: A case report. Journal of Chiropractic Medicine. 2013;**12**(4): 288-291. DOI: 10.1016/j.jcm.2013.10.001

[42] Poloni MM, Marques NP, Ribeiro Junior NV, Sperandio FF, Hanemann JAC, de Carli ML. Bell's palsy treated with photobiomodulation in an adolescent: Rare case report and review of the published literature. International Journal of Paediatric Dentistry. 2018; **28**(6):658-662. DOI: 10.1111/ipd.12424

[43] Bernal Rodriguez CG, Berlingieri Polho I, Azevedo LH, de Paula EC. Photobiomodulation therapy to treat facial paralysis of 8 years: Case report. Photobiomodulation, Photomedicine, and Laser Surgery. 2020;**38**(8):477-480. DOI: 10.1089/photob.2019.4763

[44] House JW, Brackmann DE. Facial nerve grading system. Otolaryngology–Head and Neck Surgery. 1985; **93**(2):146-147. DOI: 10.1177/019459988509300202

[45] VanSwearingen JM, Brach JS. The facial disability index: Reliability and validity of a disability assessment instrument for disorders of the facial neuromuscular system. Physical Therapy. 1996;**76**(12):1288-1298. DOI: 10.1093/ptj/76.12.1288

[46] Ross B, Fradet G, Nedzelski JM. Development of a sensitive clinical facial grading system. Otolaryngology - Head and Neck Surgery. 1996;**114**(3):380-386. DOI: 10.1016/s0194-5998(96)70206-1

[47] Nejatifard M, Asefi S, Jamali R, Hamblin MR, Fekrazad R. Probable positive effects of the photobiomodulation as an adjunctive treatment in COVID-19: A systematic review. Cytokine. 2021;**137**:155312. DOI: 10.1016/j.cyto.2020.155312

[48] Cotler HB, Chow RT, Hamblin MR, Carroll J. The Use of Low Level Laser Therapy (LLLT) For Musculoskeletal Pain. MOJ Orthopedics & Rheumatology. 2015;**2**(5):00068. DOI: 10.15406/mojor.2015.02.00068

[49] Rothschild D, Ng SY. The use of phototherapy for Bell's Palsy. In: Selected Topics in Facial Nerve Disorders. London, UK: IntechOpen; 2018. DOI: 10.5772/intechopen.81508

[50] Bello-Silva MS, de Freitas PM, Aranha ACC, Lage-Marques JL, Simões A, de Paula EC. Low- and high-intensity lasers in the treatment of herpes simplex virus 1 infection. Photomedicine and Laser Surgery. 2010; **28**(1):135-139. DOI: 10.1089/pho.2008.2458

[51] Amat A, Rigau J, Waynant RW, Ilev IK, Anders JJ. The electric field induced by light can explain cellular responses to electromagnetic energy: A hypothesis of mechanism. Journal of Photochemistry and Photobiology B: Biology. 2006;**82**(2):152-160. DOI: 10.1016/j.jphotobiol.2005.10.001

[52] Barbosa RI, Marcolino AM, de Jesus Guirro RR, Mazzer N, Barbieri CH, de Cássia Registro Fonseca M. Comparative effects of wavelengths of low-power laser in regeneration of sciatic nerve in rats following crushing lesion. Lasers in Medical Science. 2010;**25**(3):423-430. DOI: 10.1007/s10103-009-0750-8

[53] Lee J, Carpena NT, Kim S, Lee MY, Jung JY, Choi JE. Photobiomodulation at a wavelength of 633nm leads to faster functional recovery than 804nm after facial nerve injury. Journal of Biophotonics. 2021;**14**(10):e202100159. DOI: 10.1002/jbio.202100159

[54] Moriyama H, Mitsukawa N, Itoh M, Otsuka N. A view of the therapy for Bell's Palsy based on molecular biological analyses of facial muscles. The Journal of International Advanced Otology. 2017; **13**(3):414-416. DOI: 10.5152/iao.2017.3971

[55] Gavish L, Houreld NN. Therapeutic efficacy of home-use photobiomodulation devices: A systematic literature review. Photomedicine and Laser Surgery. 2018; **37**(1):4-16. DOI: 10.1089/pho.2018.4512

[56] Javaherian M, Attarbashi Moghaddam B, Bashardoust Tajali S, Dabbaghipour N. Efficacy of low-level laser therapy on management of Bell's palsy: A systematic review. Lasers in Medical Science. 2020;**35**(6):1245-1252. DOI: 10.1007/s10103-020-02996-2

[57] Hamblin MR, Nelson ST, Strahan JR. Photobiomodulation and cancer: What is the truth? Photomedicine and Laser Surgery. 2018;**36**(5):241-245. DOI: 10.1089/pho.2017.4401